PRINCIPLES OF FORENSIC MEDICINE

PRINCIPLES OF FORENSIC MEDICINE

Stephen P Robinson

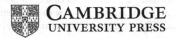

CAMBRIDGE
UNIVERSITY PRESS

CAMBRIDGE UNIVERSITY PRESS
Cambridge, New York, Melbourne, Madrid, Cape Town, Singapore, São Paulo

Cambridge University Press
The Edinburgh Building, Cambridge CB2 8RU, UK

Published in the United States of America by Cambridge University Press, New York

www.cambridge.org
Information on this title: www.cambridge.org/9780521687393

First published by Greenwich Medical Media 1996
Digitally reprinted by Cambridge University Press 2008

A catalogue record for this publication is available from the British Library

ISBN-13 978-0-521-68739-3 paperback

Every effort has been made in preparing this book to provide accurate and
up-to-date information which is in accord with accepted standards and
practice at the time of publication. Although case histories are drawn
from actual cases, every effort has been made to disguise the identities of
the individuals involved. Nevertheless, the authors, editors and publishers
can make no warranties that the information contained herein is totally
free from error, not least because clinical standards are constantly
changing through research and regulation. The authors, editors and
publishers therefore disclaim all liability for direct or consequential
damages resulting from the use of material contained in this book. Readers
are strongly advised to pay careful attention to information provided by
the manufacturer of any drugs or equipment that they plan to use.

CONTENTS

INTRODUCTION

A Police Surgeon is a registered medical practitioner, who is contracted to provide services by a particular Police Force. These services should be provided from a standpoint of total objectivity and independence. Apart from any statutory obligations, they should relate only to the clinical demands of the case in question.

These guidelines have been produced for Greater Manchester Police, for the use of their Police Surgeons.

The contents contain fact, references and opinion. The opinion is that of the author, but hopefully represents a consensus of what is considered good practice in clinical forensic medicine.

Greater Manchester Police (GMP) is the largest Constabulary Force in England, outside the Metropolitan Police Service; however, as each force in the United Kingdom is autonomous certain specific aspects of this document will be parochial to GMP and will not be relevant to other forces. Such variance will only relate to specific named forms and procedures, and the application will be just as valid to Police Surgeons in other forces, even if the documentation varies.

The Police Surgeon's work does fall into certain categories, some of which are more natural than others. For the sake of this document an arbitrary division has been devised thus:-

1. Clinical records
2. Consent
3. Disclosure
4. Statement & Report Writing
5. Fitness to be Detained
6. Fitness to be Interviewed
7. Examination in Cases of Assault
8. Examination of Victim in Cases of Sexual Assault
9. Examination of Suspect in Cases of Sexual Assault
10. The Scene of Death
11. Mental Health
12. Road Traffic Offences
13. Appendices
List of Acronyms, References and Index

It is advised that the whole document is read so that the reader can familiarise him/herself with the layout and relationship of the chapters. Most of the chapters can be read independently.

Appendicies are referrenced in the following way: Appendix 3b relates to the second appendix referred to in chapter 3.

It is intended to update these guidelines regularly, to take account of new treatment plans, changes in workload, case law and legislation.

The guidelines are meant to be advisory and not proscriptive. It appears that it would be even more difficult to achieve rigid protocols in forensic medicine, that would satisfy all the possible situations, than in other branches of medical practice. The guidelines have been well researched, and it is recommended that the advice contained is followed where applicable.

There has never been any intention that this text replaces standard textbooks or the various journals relating to clinical forensic medicine. It is meant to be a practical guide to areas which are not and could not be approached by the more academic publications. Certain aspects of the guide will not go into great depth, one example would be estimation of time since death. It is hoped that the information in the chapters that follow will however point the forensic clinician in the direction of resources for more in-depth reading.

A note about training

Clinical forensic medicine is changing rapidly. Practitioners have a duty to seek in-depth training in all aspects of the field, and particularly, but not exclusively, in the areas of medical jurisprudence in which they practise.

Continued professional development, keeping abreast of world literature and attending lectures and seminars is as important for the experienced physician as it is for the novice.

Throughout the document Police Surgeons are referred to by that title or as Forensic Medical Examiner (FME) and occasionally as Forensic Clinician. Many other titles have been considered, and this choice of usage should not be taken as an endorsement of any particular appendage, but is for consistency and ease.

If a situation is encountered which is not covered by these advisory notes, a summary of the situation clearly stating the problems encountered would be welcome by the principal author. Such information should be sent to:-

Dr Stephen P Robinson
GMP Senior Police Surgeon
Rose Cottage
Sunbank Lane
Ringway
Cheshire
WA15 0PZ

AUTHOR AND CONTRIBUTORS

Author: *Stephen P Robinson*
FAGIN Institute of Forensic Medicine
Department of Pathological Sciences
Manchester University Medical School

Contributors: *Raine El Roberts* MBE
Clinical Director
St. Mary's Sexual Assault Centre
St. Mary's Hospital
Manchester

Timothy Knowlson
FAGIN Institute of Forensic Medicine
Department of Pathological Sciences
Manchester University Medical School

Victoria Evans
Clinical Assistant
Northwest Regional Drug Dependency
Unit & Forensic Clinician

Acknowledgements

I am deeply indebted to a great number of people.

To the three mentioned on the previous page for their encouragement, input and corrections.

To Greater Manchester Police for supporting the project wholeheartedly without being at all intrusive; particularly Superintendent Kevin Hart who chaired the subcommittee overseeing the project and his team, also Chief Superintendents Trevor Barton and Glyn Morgan for their support and encouragement.

Others in alphabetical order – and I apologize for any I have missed

Dr A Campbell	Forensic Psychiatrist
Dr M Clarke	Forensic Clinician
Mr L Gorodkin	Coroner
Dr G Gudjonsson	Forensic Psychologist
Prof J Gunn	Forensic Psychiatrist
Dr J Howitt	Forensic Clinician
Dr M Knight	Forensic Clinician
Dr M Robinson	Forensic Clinician
Dr D Rogers	Forensic Clinician
Dr H Sturgess	Forensic Clinician
Dr J Tankel	Forensic Clinician
Mr A Taylor	Chief Crown Prosecutor
Mr P Taylor	Barrister
Dr M Wilks	Forensic Clinician

Other GMP police surgeons for their comments on Fitness to be Detained, and of course my wife and family who have tolerated the obsession.

1

CLINICAL RECORDS

CLINICAL RECORDS FOR POLICE SURGEONS

It is absolutely vital that FMEs keep a permanent record of their clinical findings in any work done in the forensic field.

This chapter is divided into sections. These sections will indicate:-

— The chronometry of the record **"WHEN"**

— The method of keeping **"HOW"**

— The content of the record **"WHAT"** and

— The storage of the record **"WHERE"**

WHEN

If your clinical note is going to be used in court then the record should be made at the time of the examination.

During or immediately after the contact is equally acceptable. Any delay could cast doubt on the accuracy of the record. The acceptability of a record and its contemporaneity is dealt with in more detail in chapter 4 dealing with Statements and Court.

If the record is found to be incomplete or incorrect, hours, days or even much later, and your memory of the omission or mistake is absolutely clear, then any amendment made to the record should be in a form which clearly distinguishes it from the original and from which it should be physically separate, such as on another sheet of paper. The timing of the amendment should be clearly recorded. Any additional information justifying or qualifying the changes should also be added. If a statement or report has already been submitted, or copies of the notes disclosed before the amendment is considered, then the additional material should be forwarded to the appropriate party under a fresh statement heading see Chapter 4 for statement writing.

The record should be kept for at least the natural life of the FME.

Even if the doctor has given up forensic work, it is possible that the content of the record may be called upon through the courts many years later. The recent history of miscarriages of justice (eg Kisco, Judith Ward) would indicate the necessity for the preservation of any record for at least decades. The FME has an ethical duty to the patient and the authorities who requested the examination, to preserve that record for all time.

The NHS Executive has recently issued guidance[1] on the subject of General Practice Medical Records and has recommended an increase in preservation time of the records which in broad summary is now 10 years after the patient's death. Though this directive does not relate directly to FME's records it indicates the importance placed on the long term availability of clinical records.

HOW

The written record is still the most common form of hard copy for clinical records in forensic medicine. In today's practice there are numerous other options available. Audiotape, video tape, computer discs using the various memory options available, are examples. Whatever method is used it must be remembered that the original recording is the contemporaneous note, and not a transcript! For example a hand held micro cassette recorder produces a micro-cassette of electromagnetic tape as the original record. It is that which comprises the record which must be preserved and to which one could refer in court. However, any valid document can be referred to before going into court, but contemporaneity confers the special benefit of being able to be used whilst giving evidence.

Computerised records are acceptable in civil cases[2] if that was the best form of the record and it was recorded at the time. Though a laptop computer would readily lend itself to methods of recording data, written and diagrammatic, and with the advent of digital photography, pictures as well, the system would have to be a comprehensive one to replace the standard written record. Paper free computerised records should probably only be used when the FME has such a comprehensive system.

At the moment written records are to be recommended.

They should be legible at least to the author but preferably to others as well. If medical "shorthand" is used, a legend explaining the text should be to hand, when you and the record arrive at court.

It is far better and looks more professional to use either a hard backed book or pre-prepared individual sheets.

A hard backed book is easier to store than many individual sheets of paper, and could demonstrate the contemporaneous nature of the notes by a single record's position in the book. However it is not easy or tidy to store additional material and copies of other documents, such as drug database forms or consent forms, in a hard backed book. The very nature of a bound book containing numerous records makes it difficult to preserve the confidentiality of other cases if your record is taken in as an exhibit, a circumstance which has happened to contemporaneous clinical records in the past.

Though bound books are acceptable, the recommendation is for the use of individual sheets of paper. The use of aides-memoir in the form of pre-printed sheets can be extremely helpful, though the use of comprehensive multipage booklets for every case is not advocated, when often only a small percentage of the document will be used in an individual situation. Examples of these booklets have been produced by some constabulary forces. This may raise the question as to who owns the record. **The Police Surgeon who examines the patient and makes the record has proprietorial rights of that record, and responsibility for it.**

There is no place for using torn pieces of scrap paper, or the back of constabulary stationary. It is acceptable to make additional notes on the back of copies of constabulary forms used specifically for a case, such as HO/RT/5 (see Chapter 12) in a case of blood sampling for a drink/driving offence, but in preference it is recommended that individually prepared sheets are used. These can also contain a consent form (see Chapter 2). One example of such a sheet is shown in Appendix 1a and 1b. This form has administration details on the front and standard medical history format on the back. These forms are just examples; it is advisable for individual clinicians to design a form with which they are comfortable and which can contain the appropriate information. A non specific form, similar to the ones mentioned above, is available from GMP for their Police Surgeons and is shown at Appendix 1d & 1e, however this form is not to be considered proscriptive. In addition body charts are a useful tool. Examples are shown in Appendix 1c, Charts 1-6. There are six charts in this set and all are A3 in size. The copyright belongs to the Association of Police Surgeons (APS) and they are available, to members, from the Association of Police Surgeons Office in Harrogate. FMEs may then make working photocopies from these sets.

Other similar charts are in common use, and as long as the chart is clear and simple any such pictogram could be used.

For supplies of the APS charts from which photocopies can be made write to:-

Mrs Christine Houseman
Association of Police Surgeons
18a Mount Parade
Harrogate
North Yorks
HG1 1BX

Added to the clinical notes and diagrams should be copies (photo or carbonated) of any form issued if the clinical notes are going to be complete. Thus copies of HO/RT/5, form 717 (Appendix 3c and see also Chapter 3 Disclosure), and prescriptions that are issued to prisoners or detained persons should form part of the clinical record of the patient. Though it is perfectly acceptable just to keep a record of prescriptions issued, there is nothing as accurate as a copy of the original. Self-carbonated pads with the clinician's name and professional address would be one example of fulfilling this function. The pads could also then be used for casualty referral letters or any other communication to a third party. However any letterhead with carbon paper would serve the same ends.

WHAT

The Police Surgeon's record should contain the following

- Who was seen.
- The time, date, duration and place of examination.
- At whose request the examination was made and/or the officer responsible if appropriate.
- Anyone else present at the time of examination.
- Why the examination was performed.
- The consent form for the examination.
- A history of the relevant medical condition or incident such that a professional judgement and interpretation of the clinical findings can be made.
- The clinical examination findings.
- A record/list of any samples that may have been taken.
- A record of any procedures (eg referral to Casualty/ X-ray) that may have been instituted including a copy of the referral letter.
- A copy of any instructions issued to the patient or custody officer.
- A copy of any document given in connection with the examination (eg HO/RT/5) or any prescription issued.
- Copies of any subsequent correspondence or reports connected with the case.
- If the police surgeon has been involved with another individual or scene connected with the current case, the risk of contamination (Locard's principle) should be declared and the measures taken to avoid that risk should be listed. (If such contamination could be a threat to the integrity of evidence gathering, different police surgeons should be used wherever possible).

WHERE

The storage must be secure, as for any medical record containing confidential information.

It must remain in the care of the Police Surgeon who made the record.

It must be easily retrievable, for later reference for statement construction or use in court.

Code C of the Police and Criminal Evidence Act Codes of Practice under paragraph *9C* of the notes for guidance (page 49 of the latest codes [10 April 1995]) states that the custody record must indicate where the medical practitioner has recorded his findings if they are not on the custody record.

Reference should also be made to Chapter 4 on statement and report writing.

...understanding in the case of the Police surgeon who made the examination.

It may be easily referable to their distance and surrounding circumstances, from the accused.

Court to the Plaintiff and Criminal law libraries credited to his own expense, proof will be kept for conducting the Authentic laws necessary to and to find that in a clearly engaging to inflame, so much a common understanding that, the feelings where they are none, the custody itself.

Reference should also be made to judicial environment and appeasement, the...

2

CONSENT

CONSENT BY POLICE SURGEONS

A SUMMARY

(Certain aspects of this chapter will be repeated later in this book for purposes of clarity and ease of reference).

Police surgeons are called upon to examine individuals in various circumstances.

Though largely called upon by the Police Force to whom they are contracted, they may provide services to various other agencies, eg

- Private individuals
- The Courts
- Social Services

Whatever the mechanism of the "call-out" and wherever the patient/client/prisoner is seen, the obligations re **consent** and **disclosure** are the same.

Disclosure is dealt with under a separate heading but mention is made in this document (Chapter 4).

There are three "types of contract" that Police Surgeons may have with their patients.

1. Therapeutic
2. Forensic
3. Police Complaints Authority

THERAPEUTIC

This is the usual contact and the standard doctor/patient relationship exists.

The doctor has a responsibility to treat to a standard which is acceptable by a large body of Police Surgeons and the consent is normally that of the standard "GP" type contact. This usually means that consent for the history and basic examination is virtually assumed, and written consent should be unnecessary. It does behove the doctor to follow current attitudes with a high level of patient involvement in the doctor/patient relationship.

A recent document produced jointly by the British Medical Association Ethics

Committee and the Association of Police Surgeons[3] offers similar advice but does rightly advocate written consent whenever possible.

However it must be remembered by the attending physician, particularly in the case of persons detained in custody, that his attendance may have been requested by someone other than the patient.

In that case the doctor should make it clear to the patient why the consultation has been requested and make sure that verbal consent, at least, is obtained. Obtaining verbal consent does not excuse the practitioner from documenting the exact nature of that consent.

An example may be the prisoner who has vomited. The custody officer appropriately calls out the police surgeon and acquaints the doctor with these observations. The police surgeon must inform the patient why he or she has been called unless the seriousness of the presentation indicates immediate treatment and the patient is too ill for consent to be considered. In such a case the treatment should be limited to that required for the preservation of life and the limitation of acute morbidity.

It must be remembered that the duty to a minor in the custodial situation is exactly that, as regards treatment, as exists with any caring physician. The child who has reached the age of 16 has the right to give or withhold consent (Forensic Law Reform Act - FLRA),[4] so long as that child is of sound mind. There is nothing in the FLRA precluding the child who is under 16 having the right to consent so long as the child has sufficient understanding to appreciate the examination, treatment and consequences of the illness and treatment.[5] There would be no need to wait for the parents to attend to contemplate the treatment likely to be needed from the police surgeon. The younger the child and the more serious the condition the more likely that parental consent is needed, except in the case of life threatening conditions. Indeed it is considered unlikely that a child aged 13 or less has the maturity to make a balanced judgement[6] but as youngsters are rarely kept in the custodial situation for very long, police surgeons are fortunate in being faced with difficult decisions extremely rarely, if at all, in connection with this situation. The Children Act 1989[7] comes to our aid in that it does confer the right of any person who does not have parental responsibility but does have care of the child to do what is necessary for the purpose of safeguarding or promoting the child's welfare, thus consent to immediate and necessary treatment could be given by the custody officer.

It is worth noting, however, that it is unclear in law whether or not a minor has the right to refuse treatment if it is considered absolutely necessary. This situation is not one which would apply to the acute presentation in custody, and will not be discussed here. It is an ethical and medico-legal area which should however be studied by forensic clinicians for its academic value.

The question of chaperonage should also be considered. In general terms when examining a detained person of the opposite sex a chaperone of the same sex as the patient **should** be used. It is courteous to introduce the chaperone to the patient and seek his/her approval. If the patient refuses to have the chaperone present then the doctor must carefully consider the position before commencing with any examination. It is sometimes possible to have the chaperone within sight but out of immediate earshot, and this can be acceptable to the patient who has doubts about the advisability of a non-medical person being present, particularly if that person is a police officer.

FORENSIC

A forensic examination confers no immediate health benefit to the patient. There is an argument that the examination of a victim of assault of any type, may have a therapeutic effect in the gathering of supportive evidence alone, though this could, in the long term, with the absence of a conviction, have a deleterious effect. There appears to be no research which has been done with this in mind. The immediate forensic examination does give the caring, compassionate and competent forensic clinician the opportunity for early counselling and reassurance. However the forensic examination is performed to gather evidence, for the benefit of the community, through the courts, which will support or refute an allegation in criminal proceedings. It is not made for therapeutic reasons.

The consent should be written. Though verbal consent is just as valid in theory it can never replace the evidential value of the written word. The consent should include the reasons for performing the examination[a] and also preferably include the taking of samples. Photography can be useful as an adjunct to the handwritten records and/or sketches and is extremely useful as a teaching accessory later. **If photography is considered necessary for evidential purposes then the FME should contact the Senior Investigating Officer with regard to use of the professionally trained police photographer.** The consent should include this aspect of the record as a separate item which can be deleted if inappropriate or if the consent is withheld. The use of photography,[b] for the clinical record, should be a matter between the doctor and the patient alone. Only the latter has the right to consent (and/or parent if appropriate) and only the former is fit to judge whether it would be a useful way of recording part of the clinical record or useful for forensic education. Arguments have been offered to suggest that police surgeons should not take their own photographs, as these are essentially amateur by nature. The argument progresses by suggesting that such photographs could be used adversely in any subsequent court case. Such an argument is fallacious so long as it is made clear that the photographs were only an adjunct to the written clinical records. The photograph should no

---

a. By examination I refer to the whole medical interface, including history, record keeping, clinical examination and obtaining samples.

b. By photography I also include electronic visual recording devices and not just photographic ones.

more cause problems than should sketches made by the police surgeon. There appears to be no record of any recommendation that should the police surgeon require a sketch of any injury to be made a police professional artist should be summoned.

If there is a witness to the consent, he or she could be requested to also acknowledge the consent by signing in an appropriate place. Usually, it is not appropriate for a police officer to be present at a forensic medical examination of a detained person, and there would not normally be such a witness. The doctor must, of course, consider chaperonage, and it may be that a police officer is the only person available to provide such a service. In the case of an alleged victim of sexual assault, the complainant may already have formed a secure relationship with a police officer, in which case, with the patient's consent, it would be perfectly reasonable for that officer to be present and act as a witness to the consent. The safety of the doctor has also to be considered and it may be a condition of the custody staff that an officer or officers must be close at hand if the examinee has the potential for violence against the doctor. The FME should also feel free to request such guardianship but should then document the reasons why in the clinical notes.

For the purposes of a forensic examination in the case of a suspect of an offence, the minimum age of consent should be 17.[8] Below 17 years, the consent of the parent as well as that of the child should also be sought. But please beware of acting without due consent from the appropriate authority if a "section 8[9]" is extant. This latter caveat should also apply to therapeutic examinations.

Section 8 of the Children Act 1989 defines four "orders" in Subsection (1). They are

- A contact order
- A prohibited steps order
- A residence order
- A specific issue order

It is the possibility of the 2nd and 4th of these orders which could affect the police surgeon's role.

" "a prohibited steps order" means an order that no step which could be taken by a parent in meeting his parental responsibility for a child, and which is a kind specified in the order, shall be taken by any person without the consent of the court;"

" "a specific issue order" means an order giving directions for the purpose of determining a specific question which has arisen, or which may arise, in connection with any aspect of parental responsibility for a child."

In any case it is possible that during an examination the purpose changes or evolves, or has overtones with both therapeutic and forensic implications. Unless comprehensive informed consent was obtained at the beginning, the consent of the patient should be re-assessed as soon as it becomes clear that the purpose may have altered. This would be particularly relevant in the case of a therapeutic event suddenly revealing a forensic finding of significance. An example follows.

- A prisoner complains of a headache, and the police surgeon is called. During the examination the doctor notices a soft tissue swelling at the back of the head and the detained person then says that it was caused by a police officer and he is to make a formal complaint after he is released and he would like the doctor to make appropriate records to substantiate his grievance. Having satisfied him/herself that the therapeutic situation has been dealt with, any further documentation for legal reasons must be accompanied by a re-appraisal of the consent.

A later examination for any purpose involves the re-evaluation of the consent.

POLICE COMPLAINTS AUTHORITY

When a Police Surgeon responds to a request to examine any individual, detained or not, *because* the latter has made an official complaint against a police officer, then the rules pertaining to the Forensic type examination apply. This situation is slightly more complicated and the reasons behind this are dealt with in the notes on Disclosure (Chapter 3) which follow.

GENERAL NOTES ON CONSENT

Reproduced in Appendix 2a is the consent form used by the author. This form is not proscriptive but does contain the elements which are of importance. Those items which are not valid, in the choices shown by slash marks, can be deleted.

In the space left open after "allegations of" should be put the reason given for the request. An example is a suspect or victim in a case of rape, when the word *rape* could be inserted, and the words "allegations of" left undeleted. It is important to set the scene that as a physician one is non partisan in the field of play.

The paragraph immediately before the space for signatures beginning "I also understand" is a more recent addition to the form (January 1994). The patient's attention should be drawn to this paragraph. It places the information directly before the patient that there is no absolute privilege with regard to medical consultations.

There is another area which may cause difficulty for the FME. A prisoner who is, for example, intoxicated may sign consent for disclosure at the time of the intoxication. The prudent police surgeon must carefully consider whether, when asked for disclosure at a later date, the consent would be valid. If in doubt further consent should be obtained. The test could be based on not only whether the patient understood the implications at the time but also whether the clinical record indicates that this aspect was considered and documented, and the patient understood the consequences of the consent to disclosure.

A final point to be considered is that of **duress**. The forensic clinician must be satisfied he/she was not involved in any duress regarding the consent obtained.

QUICK REFERENCE

- Is the patient a child of less than 13 years?

  Immediate necessary treatment *only*, await parental consent for anything further.

- Is the patient a child between 13 and 16?

  If the child has necessary understanding – any therapeutic measures can be taken with consent of child alone.

- Is the examinee a child under 17 and a suspect in a criminal investigation?

  Await parental consent as well as child's consent.

- Is the examinee a child under an existing section 8 of the Children Act 1989?

  Immediate and necessary treatment *only*, await guidance from the court for anything else.

- Have you got consent with regard to disclosure?

- Have you warned the examinee with regard to the non existence of privilege with regard to medical records?

3

DISCLOSURE AND CONFIDENTIALITY

DISCLOSURE BY POLICE SURGEONS

Police surgeons are called upon to examine individuals in various circumstances.

Though largely called upon by the Police Force to whom they are contracted, they may provide services to various other agencies, eg:-

- Private individuals
- The Courts
- Social Services

Whatever the mechanism of the "call-out" and wherever the patient/client/prisoner is seen, the obligations re **consent** and **section** are the same.

Consent is dealt with under a separate heading, but in this document it suffices to say that section should be covered in the consent at the start of the encounter, or wherever the "contract" changes.

There are three "types of contract" that police surgeons may have with their patients.

1. Therapeutic
2. Forensic
3. Police Complaints Authority

GENERAL INFORMATION

It must be remembered that there is no absolute privilege in the courts in the UK regarding confidentiality of a doctor/patient relationship. There is, as yet, no statutory provision regarding such confidentiality, though there is common law provision which in general leads the patient to expect confidentiality from that disclosed to the doctor in a medical situation. To access medical records, however a special procedure application has to be made to a Circuit Judge.

There is a basic medical ethic relating to confidentiality, which has been penned in various forms, dating as far back as the Hippocratic oath.[c] This ethic has been reprised in the Declaration of Geneva (as amended at Sydney 1968) thus - "I will respect the secrets which are confided in me, even after the patient has died" and also in the International Code of Medical Ethics thus "A Doctor shall preserve absolute secrecy on all he knows about a patient because of the confidence entrusted to him".

This is probably more succinctly put in the General Medical Council's (GMC) advice on Professional Conduct and Discipline. This states " Doctors therefore have a duty not to disclose to any third party information about an individual that they have learned in their professional capacity, directly or indirectly, except in the cases discussed.."[10] In October 1995 new guidance was issued by the GMC in the form of four booklets under the heading "Duties of a doctor" which gives similar advice to previous documents and should be mandatory reading for all medical practitioners.

Later paragraphs in the GMC's document discuss the situations where disclosure is acceptable, and these are covered, where relevant, in the remainder of this document.

A new booklet (May/June 1994) *Health Care of Detainees in Police Stations* has been produced jointly by the British Medical Association Medical Ethics Committee and the Association of Police Surgeons. This is available from the former at

> BMA House
> Tavistock Square
> London
> WC1H 9JP

This covers amongst other aspects of health care, advice regarding section. The information in that booklet is already included in this document but the booklet is recommended reading. This booklet is currently being updated.

THERAPEUTIC

In this area the section is now covered by statute in certain circumstances.

The main area of consideration is the Access to Health Records Act 1990 (AHRA). It must be remembered, however, that the Data Protection Act 1984 (DPA) will apply if the health record is kept on computer and is identifiable. If the records are kept on computer in such a manner the doctor has a duty to register under the DPA. The Access to Medical Reports Act 1988 could rarely apply if there was a request from an Insurance Company or Employer with regard to a patient seen for health reasons by a police surgeon.

---

c. "All that may come to my knowledge in the exercise of my profession....which ought not to be spread abroad. I will keep secret and never reveal."

The AHRA defines a "health record" as "a record made by a health professional in connection with the care[d] of that individual."[11]

The next part of the act deals with the definition of the "holder" of the health record[12] who will be the police surgeon.

Section **3** of the act defines those people who have a right to apply for access and section **3**.(1) (b) includes any person authorised in writing by the patient, which would also include a patient's solicitor.

The only exemptions that apply relate to the absence of the patient's consent, or to his/her ability to understand the nature of the application[13] when access may be wholly excluded, or to a health record made before the commencement of the Act, or relating to information which may be harmful to the patient when partial exclusion may apply.[14]

It must be remembered that there are certain clinical conditions where section is mandatory.

The FME, like any other doctor, must inform the Home Office Drugs Branch of an individual under his/her care who he considers is addicted to any of the notifiable drugs.[15]

The drugs involved are cited in the schedule to the Act and are:-

Cocaine	Hydromorphone	Oxycodone
Dextromoramide	Levorphanol	Pethidine
Diamorphine	Methadone	Phenazocine
Dipipanone	Morphine	Piritramide
Hydrocodone	Opium	

The information to be given (if known) is:-

Name	address	sex	date of birth
National Health Service number		date seen	
Name of drug.			

This information must be supplied to the Chief Medical Officer of the Home Office within 7 days of the date seen unless previously notified within the last twelve months. There is no need to notify again if such notification has been given by a **partner** or **employer** (if general practitioner employer) or fellow

---

d. Care is defined under s11. of the Act to include examination, investigation, diagnosis and treatment.

employee in same firm or a doctor on the staff of a hospital if the attendance was at the hospital.

Every individual Police Surgeon, even when working in a group, has the duty to notify.[16]

Wherever possible it is recommended that the self carbonated Drug Misuse Database forms are used (v.i.). There are Regional Research Units from whom these forms are available.

The full list of regional addresses are shown at Appendix 3b. Many of the regions use the same forms as the one referred to in the text, and these are marked with an asterisk.

These forms have 3 parts, the first (pink) is to retained and can therefore form part of the contemporaneous notes on the patient. The second (white) contains all the information as mentioned above to send to the Chief Medical Officer (CMO) of the Home Office. The last sheet (yellow) should be sent to the database office. A prepaid envelope for the database office and a prepaid addressed label for the CMO are included with the forms.

The forms satisfy confidentiality by blocking out the unnecessary data on the 2nd and 3rd sheets. A copy of the front sheet is shown at Appendix 3a.

Certain infectious diseases must be notified and these are covered by statute.[17] There are only 5 "notifiable diseases" defined under that term by the Act and those are:-

a) Cholera
b) Plague
c) Relapsing fever
d) Smallpox
e) Typhus

The usual list of common "infectious diseases" creates a second category of "diseases which are required to be notified" and are covered by Regulation 3 Schedule 1 of the Public Health (Infectious Diseases) Regulations 1988.[18]

The current list (August 1994) from Schedule 1 is shown at Appendix 3d.

It should also be remembered that there is usually a modest fee payable for notification. The form of notification is laid out in Schedule 2 of the above regulations, and such forms are available from the local Public Health Officers.

NB — The law is complicated with regard to the "infectious diseases", and should notification be contemplated and the doctor is unfamiliar with the procedure further advice should be sought. This is particularly true with regards to Acquired Immune Deficiency Syndrome (AIDS) to which only a very limited number of the sections of the 1984 Act, referred to above, apply.

One document that was used extensively and referenced above is highly recommended for further reading for any police surgeon who wishes to study further the law on communicable disease. This is:-

Communicable Disease Control - A Practical Guide to the Law for Health and Local Authorities: James T H Button - Public Health Legal Information Unit in association with Department of Health & Welsh Office. It is available at a cost of £9.25 from:-

BAPS
Health Publications Unit
DSS Distribution Centre
Heywood Stores, Manchester Road
Heywood Lancashire
OL10 2PZ

Venereal disease notification is covered by statute which also protects identification of individuals.[19] Though this Statutory Instrument relates to "officers" of Health Authorities, it sets a guideline to limited identification of patients suffering from sexually transmitted disease. A later piece of Legislation[20] extends the protection of individuals' identity to National Health Service (NHS) Trusts but does allow the passage of information to communicate to medical practitioners and for the purposes of treatment.

The greatest dilemma of confidentiality in the therapeutic interface is that, unexpectedly, the FME may be asked to provide a report or statement at a later date. If the original contact had been a therapeutic one, of apparently little medico-legal consequence, the FME may have relied on verbal and limited consent relevant to the treatment involved. In that case the FME should seek the consent of the individual in writing for such section, or respond to an order from the court if one exists. It behoves all FMEs to seek appropriate consent at the time of the original examination to cover disclosure.

The other area which causes concern is the information disseminated during the time in custody.

In GMP the form for custody fitness is the **Form 717 Greater Manchester Police – Medical Certificate.**

This form, recently re-designed, which has been copied for the sake of this document into Appendix 3c, has an upper section relating to driving and fitness to be detained. One option in this section suggests filling in a diagnosis. This should be completed with a brief phrase. This is of importance to follow-up consultations by other police surgeons, who will not have immediate access to the clinical notes made at the previous assessment (but see Chapter 5, Fitness to be Detained). It can also aid the custody officer with their degree of awareness. An example would be a detainee who was suffering from maturity onset diabetes, when that appellation could be put in the appropriate section. Though a custody officer is not a clinician, he/she will have a good lay knowledge of the risks and such information can give meaning to the other instructions written and also alert the officer to the possible consequences of changes of behaviour, or drowsiness.

The lower half of the Form 717 allows the doctor to put in free text. Here clear concise instructions relating to the care needed for that patient must be written. Examples would be the instructions for starting or continuing medication whilst in custody, and dietary information. Specific medical situations are dealt with in Chapter 5.

FORENSIC

In the case of an examination relating to the gathering of evidence either by samples or examination, the section should be obtained in the consent to include the investigating organisation – usually the police or social services. In the case of the latter, it may appropriate to include the police as a possible avenue for disclosure at the time of the examination.

It is ethically appropriate to disclose all the findings to the examinee at the end of the medical encounter.

If criminal proceedings are to be considered, though local rules (in GMP) indicate that any section of the findings writtne later should not be made to a defence solicitor without notifying the Divisional Commander, or the Crown Prosecution Service (CPS) or the department of the police representing the Police Complaints Authority (PCA), except for section 3, there should be no delay in providing such information.

There is no property in a witness (except for expert witness reports until served) and the defence has a right to see the evidence obtained, whether or not it is being served. There are no rules which forbid the defence lawyers talking to a police surgeon (or any witness), nominally called by the prosecution, and doing so in private. It is a courtesy protocol that such an approach is declared and agreed by both sides. This practice is sensible as it avoids allegations of coercion or coaching, for example.

The AHRA filled a gap left with regard to written notes compared with all types of computer record in the DPA. However, it can be argued that the wording of the AHRA indicates that it does not apply to the forensic role. If a police surgeon's record contains both health and forensic information, it would appear perfectly correct to supply only that information directly pertaining to health care if approached under the above Act. Opinion may vary on this point. It has been argued that "care" being defined as above does not require that examination, investigation or diagnosis be made for the purposes of, or in connection with, treatment.[21,22] The forensic information may be given in appropriate form (probably section 9 Criminal Justice Act 1967) and a fee charged. It should be remembered that the doctor may have to stand up in court in answer to his/her examination and comment on those findings, and even give an opinion upon them. Giving such an opinion is the duty of a professional witness and giving an opinion upon ones own findings does not immediately confer expert status on the doctor. However, as such, one would be within the bounds of reasonableness not to take on the burden of opining too far in such circumstances (see "OPINION" in Chapter 4). A copy of any statement so issued should be available for the CPS at the same time as it is provided to the defence.

In the absence of criminal proceedings, and if it is suspected that *any* civil action is contemplated by the examinee, take advice from your Medical Defence Organisation (MDO) before releasing any information. Though police surgeons are independent of the police forces who contract them and are there to serve the community and the courts above all else, it would be unprofessional and imprudent to release information to a "fishing expedition" which then resulted in a civil case against oneself or the Chief Constable, without first taking appropriate legal advice oneself. Do not be put off with indefinite advice from the MDO on the lines of "say nothing". Forensic clinicians have a duty to be totally impartial and detached from the cases they serve and not to appear to be playing a part in "protectionism".

A difficulty may arise in the case of an unconscious patient. A particular case illustrates this point.

A male was in Intensive Care in hospital after a head injury. A bloody battle had occurred involving more than two people and in which one had already died. The unconscious patient had blood stains on his skin, and he was a suspect for the alleged murder. The advice was to take swabs of the blood stains, including control swabs, and for these to be kept by the FME in a suitable freezer of his/her own. If the patient regained consciousness, consent could be sought later from the individual with regard to use of these samples.

It is possible that evidence, which would otherwise be lost, may just as easily aid the acquittal of the patient as well as the conviction, and the FME would be acting in good faith in obtaining the specimens. If consent were withheld, then the samples could be destroyed and the situation is exactly that which would have existed had the patient been conscious all the time and had not consented to the samples being obtained. If the patient died the sample should not be destroyed without confirming with the coroner that coronial jurisdiction does not require the sample.

The main pitfall with this approach is that the swabs, once obtained, are likely to be deemed "unused" material. Their production and analysis may be ordered by a court, ignoring completely the consent of the individual. This places the doctor in a dilemma. The important question to be put by the clinician to him/herself at the time is "Have I got the interest of the patient in mind when I perform this procedure"

POLICE COMPLAINTS AUTHORITY

Until July 1994 an examination performed in connection with a case of alleged police assault gave rise to a unique doctor/patient relationship. It appeared that the findings of that examination when produced in a report form could not be disclosed to another party (i.e. other than the Police Complaints Authority (PCA)) in a civil action without the courts having decided that the interests of justice overruled the Public Interest Immunity.

There is a catalogue of case law relating to this;[23] the main authority being Neilson *v* Laugharne.

There were a number of cases where disclosure was allowed, in any case, such as criminal proceedings[24] against the police officer or against the complainant.

However a recent House of Lords ruling in two cases[25] has overruled Neilson *v* Laugharne. Though Public Interest Immunity (PII) may still apply to certain documents of a Police Complaints Authority investigation, it is now no longer considered that all documents produced in such an investigation form a class of documentary evidence that should be so protected. It appears inherent in this recent judgement of Wiley and Sunderland, that medical reports are **not** covered by PII.

As long as the FMEs findings do not contain information which relates to police operational procedure, or to the identification of third parties, the doctor should be free to provide a report freely in consideration only of the consent obtained.

WHAT SHOULD BE DISCLOSED

This is a difficult question. The forensic examiner should make comprehensive notes including all that may possibly be relevant.

It may be that part of the medical record is then considered not only irrelevant but a potential source of mischief.

The FME in these circumstances must remember that he or she is party to only one aspect of a case.

There may be items which the FME does not wish to disclose. An example may be previous sexual history from a complainant. Sexual intercourse with a male other than the one accused only hours before *must* be included in the findings as such a situation may have great significance to the interpretation of the scientific evidence. The time scale in this example can be arbitrary. In the principal authors opinion seven days should be the minimum dividing line[e] before an FME considers excluding the section of such information with regard to a previously sexually active female.

The example above is often not the case and previous sexual history may not be considered to be relevant to the case in question. If that is so, such "confidential" knowledge need not be disclosed at the time, but its existence should be declared along with the opinion of the FME concerning its irrelevance and with a claim of Public Interest Immunity. It may then be left for the judge to decide whether the evidence can be looked at in court, initially in the absence of the jury, if so requested by an expert advising the other side.

Hard and fast rules cannot easily be made to safeguard the disclosure of material

---

e. NB Chapter 8 should be read with regard to the recovery of genetic material.

that is relevant and only that material, and each case must be judged on its own merits.

FMEs cannot become judge and jury and must serve the judicial system...warts and all!

QUICK REFERENCE

- Check consent form to determine for whom information disclosure permission was granted.

  Write report for only those persons indicated by the consent.

- Was informed consent received for disclosure?

  Write to patient to request section consent.

- Is there confidential information in your notes which you believe is irrelevant to the subject in question?

  Omit this other information, write a covering letter indicationg its presence and claim Public Interest Immunity from disclosure.

4

STATEMENT, REPORT WRITING THE WITNESS STATEMENTS

STATEMENTS

Statements and reports are here treated in the same manner.

In general the use of the word "statement" in clinical forensic terms refers to a document produced in terms that are acceptable to a criminal court in a form as laid down by section 9 of the Criminal Justice Act 1967. This act allows for evidence to be read out in court and to be treated with the same weight and value as if the evidence had been given in person. Such evidence can only be offered to the court if counsel for both sides agree that the contents are acceptable.

Reproduced here in Figure 4.1 is the appropriate paragraph that must be appended to a report (in England & Wales) for it to be in an acceptable form to satisfy presentation in court. Besides including and signing this declaration, each individual page must be signed also.

The FME producing a report, whether it is in "section 9" form or not, owes a duty to produce a document that is clear, concise and understandable to a non medically trained person. Subject to the "section 9" declaration, no distinction will be made between reports and statements.

STATEMENTS OF WITNESS

(C.J. Act 1967, s9; M.C. Rules 1981, r.70)
(Magistrates Courts Act 1980 s102)

Statement of Dr . . . .

Age of witness: date of birth . . . .

This statement (consisting of .... pages each signed by me), is true to the best of my knowledge and belief and I make it knowing that, if it is tendered in evidence, I shall be liable to prosecution if I have wilfully stated in it anything which I know to be false or do not believe to be true.

Dated the ....

Signed..

Figure 4.1 — "section 9" Declaration

In a civil case the format differs. It should be produced without the above declaration.

The structure of a medico-legal report can be broken down into a simple protocol. The order of inclusion of the various components is not critical except where the sequence of events being described is itself of significance.

Two examples are shown

1. *If the examination findings and procedures are described in an examination of a victim of an alleged rape, it is a common, but not proscriptive, practice to describe these before listing samples taken. The samples may however be taken contemporaneously with parts of the examination and it is helpful if this could be shown. Thus if the perineum were cleansed, it is worthwhile indicating that this was done after taking the perineal swab and before the internal vaginal swab, rather than expecting the court to assume such a sequence.*

2. *In the above, or any alleged assault, it is normal medical practice to take a history, and this is referred to in Chapter 1 under the subheading of What. It may be that having taken a history and proceeding to the examination, a positive sign is discovered which does not fit in with the information already gathered from the examinee. It is sound clinical practice to ask the latter if he/she can account for that finding. When this information is reproduced in the report, it should be clear which information was offered spontaneously and which was offered later as a response to the examiner's question.*

Please note that "Expert Reports" are not being considered in this document, though much of this advice applies equally to such reports.

CONTENT

The information that should be included is shown here in Table 4.1.

METHOD OF STATEMENT WRITING

The statement should be written by the doctor producing the report. The practice of dictating the statement to a third party such as a police detective creates another link in the chain that may produce unintentional inaccuracies.

If possible the statement should be typed. Even if the author of a report possesses a beautiful hand, which for a doctor appears unlikely, a typeface is still easier to read.

Who you are	
What you are	eg Police Surgeon X Division Downtown Police
Length/depth of experience	
What your qualifications are	medical, legal and scientific qualifications only – they should be in long hand form eg Bachelor of Medicine and not M.B.
Whom you examined	
When you did the examination	
What was the declared reason for the examination	
What consent was obtained	include record of any consent that was withheld
Where the examination took place	
Who else was present	
What the relevant presenting history was	
What were your clinical findings – general and specific forensic	negative findings should also be included, eg "there was no bruising visible on the back" Please see Chapter 2 on section
What samples were taken	see later section of examination of victim (Chapter 8)
What treatment if any was given (if relevant)	
A summary of your findings if at all complex or numerous	
A reasonable conclusion to explain the results of your history and examination	This is explained in more detail below under the subheading of **"opinion"**
To whom and when you passed any specimens	to prove continuity of evidence

Table 4.1

Easy access to word processing allows the Police Surgeon to prepare the statement and edit it until a satisfactory structure is achieved. It should be prepared after careful thought about content and structure.

Further benefits of word processing include saving the standard inclusions, such as the "section 9" declaration, and the individual's personal details, to speed the production of the statement.

Statements should be produced expeditiously, when requested, not only to ease the administration for the justice departments of the Police Force, but also and more importantly, not to delay the progress to trial for the accused, who may well be languishing on remand.

The FME should keep a copy, for cross reference, but this should not be referred to whilst giving evidence without the leave of the court (see Hearsay below). It is advisable for the clinician to refresh his/her memory by reading the statement before going into court.

TERMINOLOGY

A repeated plea from the legal profession is for doctors to use plain English.

Any medical term should always be accompanied by an appropriate lay word or phrase.

Such translations can be included contemporaneously in the document or listed in a glossary. The former appears to be customary.

What is not consistent is whether the scientific or lay word is the substantive one with the other following in parenthesis. One advantage of using the medical term substantively is the maintenance of accuracy. The lay term may be chosen as an illustrative one. An example could be *"haematoma (swollen bruise)"*. The lay term in this illustration is not particularly accurate, but does describe the finding, whereas haematoma has a specific medical meaning.

Accuracy of terminology is also pre-eminent.

There may be justifiable variations of understanding about certain words. Petechiae have been described as a haemorrhage into the skin of less than 1 mm[26] or ≤2 mm,[27] whereas the former reference of these two would class 2 mm diameter haemorrhages as purpura. It is important that the forensic clinician decides which definition is acceptable to him/her and uses it consistently. The example given above is of little, if any, consequence in the interpretation of injuries.

The use of "laceration" for a cut to the skin caused by a sharp object is as deplorable as it is incorrect. In due course it may contribute to a miscarriage of justice and/or expose the doctor who casually used a term wrongly to professional embarrassment. Charges of assault commonly revolve around the use or not of a sharp weapon. The use of the terms incision and laceration may be critical in such cases.

An example is given:-

A fight occurs between two young adult males.

The complainant suffers a wound to the bottom lip, inferior to the vermillion border, with a smaller internal wound inside the bottom lip in the same area.

The defendant is accused of stabbing the "victim" with a pocket knife, the two wounds being interpreted as entry and exit wounds of the blade.

As such a complex of wounds could be caused by a knuckle lacerating the outside of the lip, and causing a crush laceration of the inner aspect against the cusp of a tooth, the accurate description of the wound may be critical. It is of course also vital to describe any ancillary injuries such as tooth damage, incisions or scratches on the gum, bruises etc.

Another area of contention is the description, in detail, of injuries or lesions. This area is dealt with in full detail in Chapter 7.

SEMANTICS

This is a further area of contention. The terms used everyday by physicians such as acute and chronic may be understood by the non-medical person, but not in the same way as was meant by the medic. Thus evidence may be given at length, in a relaxed and thoroughly professional manner, and the doctor leaves the court (or is not present, the "section 9" statement having been read). The judge, jury and counsel are left with an understanding of the medical matters in the case totally different from that which was intended by the doctor.

An example is given here from the lecture given by Crown Prosecution Service to North-West Police Surgeons Development Training Course 18 February 1994.

In a real statement, used as an example, the doctor had used the words " he denied using illicit drugs..." as part of his summary of the medical history of the examinee. The Crown Prosecutor leading the session voiced her opinion that "denied" was a poor choice of word, as the doctor gave no indication to indicate why he knew the individual was using illicit drugs. That the doctor involved, as well as the other assembled medics, all accepted the use of this particular phrase as standard medical practice to show that to a question about the use of illicit drugs, the person had answered "no", and that there was no slant, weight or any other opinion inherent in the phrase, was futile if the lay person would understand something different. Here the Crown Prosecutor had assumed that this particular structure of words had indi-cated a refutation by the examinee of a practice assumed by the doctor to be part of the examinee's profile and about which the police surgeon had issued a challenge.

The fault in the above illustration lies with the medics. No assumption should be made by police surgeons that everyday words used by them in practice, which are not properly classified as technical words (see terminology above), can be used casually in an evidential manner.

HEARSAY[28]

Including in a statement, or voicing in court, that which is considered hearsay is always a danger and one of which the FME, or any clinician, should be aware.

The rule against hearsay is encapsulated thus:-

"An assertion other than one made by a person while giving oral evidence in the proceedings is inadmissible as evidence of any fact asserted."[29] This applies to any kind of assertion whether by mouth, writing or gesture, eg a nod.

The rule will be strictly applied.

This rule does influence what the FME includes in the statement (or in evidence).

An example follows.

> In the case of an alleged rape, the complainant tells the doctor that the assailant held a knife point to her throat and said " I know what I am doing I have done it before".

> In the doctor's statement, it is right and proper to include the history declared by the examinee of having the knife held against her throat, as this may directly relate to the clinical findings on examination. The assertion of having "done it before" may be hearsay and the doctor should not be surprised to have that statement square bracketed. However it should still be included. This is discussed below.

In the above case the prosecution may want to adduce the spoken evidence as a matter of its cause and effect on the state of mind of the alleged victim, in which case it may be allowed. It is unlikely to be allowed if it were being introduced to "prove" the fact of the other assault.

Certain declarations made by the complainant may be admissible, under some circumstances. The doctor on quickly seeing an alleged victim shortly after an alleged sexual offence may give particulars of the complainant, which relate to the charge against the defendant, not as proof of the allegation complained of, but as evidence of consistency of the conduct of the complainant as exhibited by her testimony.

A further exception to the hearsay rules may occur which can affect the FME's statement.

Under the rule of Res Gestae,[30] evidence of words used by a person may be admissible in that they from part of the transaction (the assault for example) subject to legal proceedings. In the case of alleged rape, and early declaration and examination by a forensic clinician, the highly distressed complainant may make utterances to the doctor which can safely be regarded as a true reflection of what she is experiencing because of the trauma. Such utterances may be allowed to be given by the physician.

If there is doubt, spoken evidence should be included anyway. The doctor should not be offended if he/she later finds that inclusion "square-bracketed" out of the statement. Such an occurrence would suggest that the legal profession did not consider that evidence to be a justifiable exception to the hearsay rules.

It is conceivable that an FME being part of the investigation team, may make a record of something stated by a complainant which later may be admissible, even though it would otherwise constitute hearsay, if the patient died, or is unfit to give evidence or who, through, fear does not give oral evidence.[31] The court has the right to decide whether justice will be better served by introducing it.[32] The court must have regard to nature, source, relevance and authenticity of the statement and it therefore behoves the police surgeon to keep the clinical forensic record as pristine and legible as possible.

There are further exceptions to the hearsay rule which make fascinating reading for the interested student but which do not directly affect the production of evidence by the FME and will not therefore be included here.

ORAL EVIDENCE

The rules pertaining to statement writing also apply to giving oral evidence, with the exception that there is less time to think during the latter.

The old adage of "Dress up, Stand up, Speak up and Shut up" still reigns.

There exists a basis of expectation that the professional man or woman will look the part. That the quality of evidence given does not depend on twinset and pearls or shirt and tie is irrelevant. The prejudices of the jury and justices should be recognised and catered for. The forensic witness is not there to make a political or sociological point. He/she is there to aid the court in the administration of justice. Suits and ties and smart skirts or dresses or suits worn according to the traditonally accepted mode for your gender should be the norm.

Be prepared, locate your clinical records in advance.

Arrive at court in plenty of time if possible.

You may be allowed to refresh your memory from your statement before going into court. This should be done to link the form and structure of your statement with the clinical notes from which it was made. The statement is usually more succinct and ordered than the clinical notes, but the evidence must be given by referral to the latter.

The FME will be allowed to refer to the contemporaneous clinical notes made at the time of the examination whilst giving evidence. He/she will also be allowed to give evidence from memory. Care must be taken where this varies from the clinical notes and the FME should be certain that no confusion has arisen with other cases. Considering the time it takes to come to trial, it is quite possible that the doctor has seen many hundreds of cases subsequent to the one in question, and any confusion by the doctor which can be elicited by counsel could invalidate the value of the clinical evidence.

The rules by which a witness is allowed to refresh memory are encapsulated in the case of R *v* DaSilva (1990 1 All ER).

If the contemporaneous notes are lost it may be possible to refer to the statement. The judge in a criminal trial has a discretion to permit a witness to refresh his memory even after beginning to give evidence.

For this benefit to be given the judge be satisfied that:

1. The statement was made whilst the events recorded were fresh even if not contemporaneous.

2. The witness can no longer recall the events in question because of the lapse of time since the event.

3. That the witness did not read the statement before going into the witness box.

4. That the witness wishes to read the statement before continuing.

The witness may then be allowed to refer to the statement in or out of the witness box, but in either case must do so without communication, and on resuming evidence the statement must be removed from him.

If the statement were made immediately after the examination, it could be considered to be contemporaneous, though any discrepancy between the clinical notes and the statement would increase the potential for doubt as to accuracy. A statement should include everything that is appropriate to ease the course of justice but should be a considered and carefully constructed document, and it does not lend itself to hurried preparation.

The question may arise as to contemporaneity of a document or statement, and it may be argued that there is no hard and fast rule as to when the witness may be allowed to refresh his/her memory. It is generally accepted that when a long time has elapsed between making a statement, fairly soon, but not contemporaneously, after the events, the witness should be allowed to refresh his memory from the statement before giving evidence.

With regard to professional medical witnesses the courts are often very accommodating in allowing reference to a statement, and in many cases will actually draw the statement into the examination, or more likely cross-examination. It is important that the form and content of the statement stands scrutiny in public.

Posture in the witness box is also important. The witness may be asked if he/she wishes to sit. The choice is open, but do not sit without being invited so to do. There is no need to sit or stand rigidly to attention, but it is important to stand or sit without slouching or leaning. Such a posture not only makes it easier to project the voice but also adds to the professionalism of the testimony.

Before reaching the witness box the professional witness should have rehearsed a number of things.

1. Whether the oath or affirmation is to be taken, and if the former, on which deity or authority the oath will be sworn. If it is more comfortable to recite the appropriate words from memory or from the printed cards, try and speak to the Court Clerk, prior to giving evidence to agree the procedure in your particular case.

2. A verbal version of your profile, including who and what you are, your experience and qualifications. It may be that at the beginning of the examination in chief, counsel will lead you through this, but you may just be asked to tell the court who you are. A concise rehearsed passage will immediately indicate that you are professionally prepared and will forewarn the jury that your testimony will be in a similar state of health.

One difficulty in court is deciding to whom one should speak. It should be the "judges". In a crown court that includes the jury who judge the facts and in the magistrates court, the bench.

Even experienced expert witnesses can find themselves entering into an exclusive dialogue with the counsel asking questions, and that should be avoided.

One simple aid to achieve this has been suggested at the Expert Witness Seminar run by Bond-Solon in London. Their suggestion is to stand with feet firmly pointing towards the judge. On being asked a question by counsel the body can be partially rotated to present a receptive face towards the advocate, and on responding the natural position can be resumed, the body swinging back towards the judge. The limitations of these relatively small movements will usually mean that the response to the question is projected somewhere between the judge and jury, hopefully satisfying both their needs.

The voice should be projected, with an increase in volume but not tone if possible.

Due consideration should be given before answering, and the answer delivered in plain English in as concise and as meaningful a manner as possible. As in statement writing use non specialist language to translate technical terminology.

If a SWOT analysis[f] was done on being a witness there may be a tendency to see every question as a Threat, when in fact each should be considered an Opportunity. The police surgeon is there to serve justice; questions should be answered truthfully. Do not try to bias the answers to fit in with a prejudicial view of the court case. It is for the jury to decide the outcome (or the bench).

Barristers are trained for the job, do not underestimate them, if it is not possible to answer a question simply, say so.

Double questions are a frequent weapon of the advocate, they require clarification or two answers. If possible give the hidden answer first and the prompted one second; an example follows.

---

f. SWOT - an analysis of any situation into the areas of Strengths v Weaknesses and Opportunities v Threats.

In a case of alleged assault which actually involved an argument between two women, the complainant was the only one examined. The defendant maintained that she had suffered a minor black eye, but as the whole affair was a mutual quarrel, she did not seek medical aid as no treatment was needed. The injuries to the complainant were minimal.

The question asked was thus "you have seen the injuries suffered by the complanant, haven't you doctor, and without doubt she came off worse in the exchange". A full answer should include the fact that as the accused was not examined at the time no comparison can be made but, yes you did see the complainant's injuries which you have described,

Other apocryphal examples are shown below and it must also be recognised that questions are sometimes phrased as statements; failure to answer plainly may be an opportunity to the advocate.

"wasn't it at 4 o'clock in the morning doctor when you were tired?"

"didn't the examination only take 20 minutes doctor? you were obviously in a hurry"

"the examination took nearly 2 hours doctor didn't it? you must have been unsure of your findings" (Note that the second "question" in this example was also phrased as a statement).

It is unusual for a competent professional medic to be pressurised in the witness box. If undue pressure is being felt then an appeal to the justices in the case to allow the evidence to be given fairly will usually achieve the necessary relief. It is important however to concede a point which has a right to be adduced.

In most cases the police surgeon as a professional witness will not be party to the whole procedings. It is not appropriate to start on a monologue introducing items which are irrelevent to the way that the case is evolving. When the various stages of the examination are finished the doctor should then stop speaking (hence "shut up"). The one exception relates to the doctor being left with a feeling that the facts that were being introduced had been done so unfairly, or that a particular relevant question concerning facts already covered was not asked. It is the responsibility of the professional witness to bring the judge's attention to this problem. This may result in the jury being expelled whilst a point of law is discussed. The responsibility of whether or not the presumed omission is corrected has been passed on to the court and the FME will have behaved properly and fairly.

OPINION

The question of giving an opinion is a thorny one.

The police surgeon is a professional witness, and as such the court has the right to expect the medic to give a presentation of the appropriate "history", "examination" and "diagnosis".

The last of these constitutes the opinion in a forensic case.

Giving an opinion or interpretation of ones own findings in the light of the history given at the time of the examination, or in the light of an alternative aetiology presented in court is part of the duty of a professional witness. Such duty does not carry the appelation to convert the witness into an expert.

Early in these guidelines the caveat of "opining too far" was referred to. The professional witness who is asked to go further than considering only his/her own findings and is asked to look at other clinical or scientific documents is then being asked to give an expert opinion. The doctor should not permit him/ herself to be pressurised into opining on such material without the time to give it due consideration and thought. Such consideration of alternative medico-scientific material is asking, of the doctor, an expert's countenance, and the doctor has a right to be expected to be treated as such.

Extreme caution is advised to any doctor who accepts such a responsibility, to ensure that they have the appropriate qualifications and experience to complete the task. The doctor who can say quite simply that a certain topic is beyond or without their experience, does a favour to the court and the forensic profession. He/she also strengthens the acceptability of those areas on which they are prepared to opine.

5

FITNESS TO BE DETAINED

FITNESS TO BE DETAINED

The booklet *Health Care of Detainees in Police Stations* reported jointly by the British Medical Association (BMA), Ethics Committee and the Association of Police Surgeons and available from the BMA should be mandatory reading for all police surgeons.

The request by a custody officer to see if a prisoner is fit to be detained is probably the commonest problem a police surgeon encounters. Most cases are relatively straightforward but some can pose difficult problems. Occasionally the surgeon will be called to court to assess a case or to see individuals who are assisting the police but who are not under arrest.

In all cases the FME is duty bound:-

1. To practise good medicine and treat all persons with courtesy and respect

2. To obtain appropriate consent and explain to the patient the implications of the examination (see Chapters 2 & 3)

3. To respect confidentiality within the constraints of personal safety and public duty

4. To provide proper instructions to the police

   4.1 To enable them to care for the patient

   4.2 To advise the police about potential bio-medical hazards

These are difficult criteria to fulfill and at times may appear to present great conflict. The source of prevention of this conflict is the maintenance of high levels of communication and professional integrity, wherever possible.

This chapter will deal with the detainee in custody, but the advice is just as relevant for the other areas where fitness to be detained is the issue.

It is now common for police surgeons to be requested to assess whether a detainee is fit to be interviewed and this is dealt with in the next chapter.

GENERAL INFORMATION

There are various conditions with which the police surgeon may be faced:

1. The police surgeon is called because of the requirements of the Police and Criminal Evidence Act 1984 (PACE).
2. Existing disease, with or without medication
3. Detainees exhibiting substance abuse
4. Observed signs, injuries or abnormalities of behaviour requiring assessment.

With regard to the last of these, abnormalities of behaviour may indicate a psychiatric problem and this subject is dealt with in Chapter 11.

There is no intention of this advice becoming a large tome of internal medicine. It will however approach the subject from a general point of view and also focus on a few common conditions which may cause problems.

PROCEDURES

Discussion with custody officer

On arrival at the police station it is imperative to discuss the case with the Custody Sergeant. This establishes:-

- How or why the person is detained
- What the custodian is concerned about
- What questions need to be answered, i.e. fit to be detained, fit for interview, disposal
- What are the time constraints and any other problems faced by the custody.

It is also sensible to discuss the case with the arresting officer, if possible, to hear the circumstances of the arrest and the reason for detention. This enables one to have a clearer idea of the avenues of disposal available, i.e. home circumstances, relatives at home, etc.

It is then important to decide where you are going to see the patient/prisoner. It is usually appropriate to see them in the medical room. Violent, aggressive detainees or those with a degree of stupor are often best seen where they are, either in the cells, or holding rooms. The Custody Officer's opinion must be taken into consideration, particularly with potentially violent patients as he/she has responsibility for the safe running of the whole custody suite including other detainees. There is no room, however, for the abrogation of the FME's clinical responsibilities.

Any instructions given about the care necessary should be written. This may be done on the custody record or on special forms, designed for the purpose (see Appendix 3c for an example). The police surgeon should keep a copy. If a separate form is used, then the custody record should indicate that, as well as referring to the medical record being kept in the possession of the surgeon. This will then satisfy section 9 C of the Codes of Practice of PACE (see page 10 "WHERE").

It is important for the police surgeon to be familiar with the conditions of care and treatment demanded by PACE and should read the Codes of Practice (The Codes). A new edition of The Codes came into effect on the 10 April 1995.

If the police surgeon is relinquishing responsibility for a patient who is likely to need follow up, that surgeon should ensure that the doctor taking over any responsibility has been informed of all the relevant factors. Practitioners in a regular rota may have developed a reliable system for the dissemination of such information amongst themselves, but in all other cases written instructions should be left in a sealed envelope and marked for the attention of Medical Practitioners only. The custody staff should be informed that, were the patient to be moved to another custody area, the sealed communication along with a copy of the care instructions, if any, must go with the detainee and not be left solely on his custody record in that station.

Introduction

It is courteous and good practice to greet the prisoner and the relatives with the same courtesy that would be extended to any other patient. Not everybody in custody is a hardened cynical detainee. Some prisoners are not reassured by claims of independence but many are. It is helpful to explain the speciality of legal medicine and the independent role, and that clinical needs will be met irrespective of their problems with society.

They may wish to call their own doctor, but it should be pointed out that the latter has no obligation to attend and a fee may be payable.

They should be informed that there is always a lack of Absolute Privilege and that anything said may have to be to disclosed if so ordered by a judge in court.

Obtain the appropriate consent (see Chapter 2).

Some examinations require authority other than the doctor/patient consent. Such are examinations for **Intimate Samples** and those for **Intimate Searches**. The former is dealt with under Examination of the Suspect in Sexual Offences (see page 118) and the latter is dealt with later in this chapter (see page 73).

History

Take a standard medical history. It must be remembered however that the patient in custody may have a different agenda from that classically met in patients in standard practice. The use of leading questions may be hazardous. The story should be written as the detainee tells it; this helps with doctor/patient confidence.

It can be of value, but is not proscriptive, to use a basic proforma for the history and details. It is important to elucidate the past medical and surgical histories (see Chapter 1 & Appendices 1a-e). There are occasions when family history and social history are going to be significant and these aspects should not be overlooked. It is also important to record the use of prescribed and non-prescribed drugs. In many cases it is important to note the intake of alcohol over the previous 24 hours and when the prisoner last ate, drank and slept.

In the case of prescribed drugs, it is necessary to take a detailed history of who prescribed them, when they were last taken and if that day's doses have been taken and at what time. It is also necessary to record information arising from this for the custody officer and say exactly what tablets are needed, the doses and at what times. It is useful to record the GP's name and telephone number and the name of any consultant seen. The problem of illicit drugs is dealt with in the sub-section on the drug addict later in this chapter. It is useful to then ask if the detainee has anything else he wishes to discuss or needs. Specific aspects of history taking are dealt with under each section later in these guidelines.

Common sense has to prevail in deciding whether a prisoner with a defined condition is fit to be kept in cells. A good guideline is, if you were in general practice would you be happy to keep this patient at home or does he need hospital admission. Police officers are not trained nurses and can only perform basic tasks of nursing and should not be expected to carry out the more sophisticated observations.

In all the following situations it is safer to refer to hospital if in doubt. A death in police cells is taken very seriously and investigated like a murder enquiry. It may reveal that a patient received treatment at a level less than reasonable. Criminal prosecution could follow.

Prescribing medicine

Any detainee needing medication should be prescribed enough medication for his stay in custody. This is done on a private prescription and paid for by the police.[33]

If the detainee is to be detained for longer than 7 days, it is sensible for the medication to be reviewed at the end of this period and a further prescription issued if necessary.

Naturally the patient's condition may indicate earlier review, and the FME should then set the review period sooner to satisfy clinical need alone. Such schedules do not, of course, exclude earlier review if so requested via the custody officers.

The medication, dose and frequency of dose, or preferably specific times the medication is to be given, should be **written out** for each patient and given to the custody officer. This information should be included in the care instructions mentioned above.

SPECIFIC CONDITIONS

Heart disease

Most patients seen with heart disease are well controlled and on regular medication and present no problems.

The most difficult complaint to assess is that of chest pain. It is obviously important to decide whether it is cardiac or has some less life-threatening cause.

Most commonly a patient will be seen with a chronic condition such as angina, cardiac failure or a stable arrhythmia such as atrial fibrillation. In these cases the regular medication can be continued and prescribed in the normal way and the custody record annotated with drug dosage and the times they should be given. Simple advice can be given such as, please ring me if the patient gets worse, i.e. has chest pain, becomes breathless or is sweating.

The problems will arise with chest pain of a cardiac type and differentiating angina from infarction. The police surgeon must take a detailed history of the type of pain and record this on the notes. He/she must record the clinical examination of the heart and blood pressure and pulse rates and any evidence of cardiac failure. The basic values apply as in general practice and referral to hospital is indicated if in any doubt and a letter should be sent with the patient.

In cases where medication is needed, it should be prescribed in the doses and at the times that the detainee would normally take it outside custody. If the detainee is on symptom led medication such as a nitrate, he should be allowed to keep that in his cell unless there is a specific reason not to. Doubt as to the identity of the medication, or regular abuse of any medication are examples of where greater care of freedom to access of therapy is needed.

Epilepsy

The approach here is similar to that of cardiac disease. If you would not be happy to manage a patient at home then hospital referral is safer.

Most epileptics seen in police custody are well controlled and know their own disease well. However, many prisoners do not take their medication as prescribed and some have a high incidence of fits.

The history is important and should elucidate:

- The type of epilepsy & the type or frequency of fits
- When the prisoner last had a fit
- The medication taken in detail
- When the last dose was taken
- What doses are necessary for that day and subsequent days in custody

It is felt that one self limiting fit in custody is acceptable but a prisoner having more than one fit needs hospital review. Similarly if the fit is the first ever, then this needs hospital investigation as one would in general practice. Police officers are capable of immediate first aid and should be instructed to put the patient in the recovery position and inform the doctor.

It is worthwhile recording clearly the type of Epilepsy.

Epilepsy is a group of syndromes, they constitute "a chronic brain disorder of various aetiologies characterised by recurrent seizures due to excessive discharge of cerebral neurones."[34]

The epilepsies can be classified in a number of ways. The International League Against Epilepsy (ILEA) has produced a classification[35] based on the clinical seizure type and the ictal and post ictal EEG. As the police surgeon does not have recourse to sophisticated tertiary investigations, and often has little history from the patient and none available from previous doctors, the seizure type classification can be simplified thus:[36]

Seizure Type	Characteristics
1 Partial Seizures	
1.1 **Simple**	
1.1.1 focal origin (may be motor, sensory, autonomic or psychic)	
1.1.2 restricted to one hemisphere	
1.1.3 no disturbance of consciousness	
1.2 **Complex**	
1.2.1 focal origin	
1.2.2 involves both hemispheres	
1.2.3 consciousness is disturbed	
1.3 **Secondary Generalised**	
1.3.1 focal origin (not necessarily obvious)	
1.3.2 disturbance of consciousness?	
1.3.3 tonic–clonic fit (usually)	
2 Primary Generalised Seizures	
2.1 **Tonic**	
2.2 **Tonic–Clonic**	
2.3 **Absence** (= Petit Mal, which is an EEG diagnosis)	
2.4 **Myoclonic**	
2.5 **Atonic**	

It can be extremely difficult to differentiate between Generalised Seizures.

The importance of attempting to make a diagnosis may extend beyond immediate treatment. Automatisms do occur particularly in some complex partial seizures, and recognising such a diagnosis could save much police time, in for example a shoplifting offence. Of course the presence of epilepsy per se does not exclude criminal activity.

The decision about treatment is difficult. Some epileptics in custody exhibit chaotic treatment compliance. If there is also a personality disorder and/or substance abuse problems as well, the patient may be totally unreliable as a witness to his medication schedule. The claim that the patient is on oral Temazepam or Diazepam as an anti-epileptic should be treated with disbelief. It may be that an oral benzodiazepine (the BNF recommends Clobazam) is used as an adjunct to epilepsy with an associated anxiety state, and in that case the treatment will probably need to be continued. The decision about treatment with anxiolytics is dealt with under the sub-section dealing with substance abuse (v.i.), so will not be repeated here. The only benzodiazpine used as a long term anticonvulsant is Clonazepam, which may be used in all forms of seizure[37] but particularly in Absence attacks and Myoclonus.[38]

Other problems have to be addressed. Missing a single dose of anticonvulsant medication whilst in custody overnight, should make little difference. Many anticonvulsants have a long half life, but both Carbamazepine and Valproate have a short half life of about 12 hours. These drugs are best given in divided doses, and to avoid side effects can be administered up to four times/day. Prescribing doses of these drugs in such divided doses is unlikely to cause any side effects. It could be extremely risky to miss medication if the epilepsy is brittle. The only problem drug from the aspect of toxicity is Phenytoin. Phenytoin is subject to saturation state kinetics and it is theoretically possible, if misled by a patient, to induce significant toxicity if the patient claims to be on a nominally high dose which is continued or increased, particularly if detained in custody, or remanded to police cells for an extended time. The habit, exhibited by some patients seen in the custody situation, of bolting all and every drug in their possession, when the police officer knocks on their door prior to arrest, can further complicate matters.

With all anticonvulsants, if the patient is in custody for an extended period of time, serum levels should be obtained. Now, with the establishment of Hospital trusts, this may involve negotiations for payment of the blood test, but administrative complications should not obstruct clinical management. Most such cases are likely to be Remand Patients.

The custody record must be clearly written and annotated with the name of tablets and the time that doses must be given.

Diazepam is still the drug of choice for status epilepticus and can be administered intravenously or rectally. It is useful to carry rectal diazepam for use in a prisoner who is fitting in the cells.

Any patient who has needed parenteral anticonvulsant therapy for status epilepticus, whilst in custody, even if conscious post-ictally, needs referral to hospital.

Diabetes

Non-insulin dependent diabetics can be managed in custody with little problem. The only likely complication could be hypoglycaemia, if tablets are taken and food is not provided. However, this is unlikely under PACE rules.

The history should include any complications that are present, the name and dosage of tablets and the time at which the tablets are due. Recommendations for feeding should be conveyed to the custody officer.

It is easy for blood sugar to be measured "in the field" using any of the commercial testing sticks, and no police surgeon should be without the means to take such a measurement. The use of an electric meter to give an accurate digital read-out is neat, probably confidence building, and may show subtle changes in sequential measurements. These meters are inexpensive, but are not absolutely necessary, as a clinically reliable reading may be taken by visual comparison with the colour chart on the container. If a meter is used the clinician needs to take responsibility for any standardisation needs of the equipment. **Ideally, every diabetic staying in custody should have at least one blood sugar measured.** This may be waived if the patient is clinically well, non-insulin dependent, and only going to be in custody for a short period, say less than four hours.

The insulin dependent diabetic is more difficult to control in custody. Any diabetic who is unstable, either with hypo or hyperglycaemia, needs hospital assessment and sometimes in-patient care. Once stabilised they could be returned to police custody.

There is also a need to consider the particular circumstances of the arrest, such as recent pursuit or substance abuse.

There is the possibility for a prisoner to overdose or under-dose himself on purpose to cause problems. Ideally, the surgeon should supervise the patient drawing up and administering his insulin on the first occasion in custody to satisfy his/her need to know that the patient is competent.

Once again, clear instructions can be left to police officers about changes in condition, i.e. pallor, sweating, confusion etc.

Every detainee who is a declared or suspected diabetic should have at least one blood sugar estimated by the Police Surgeon at the time of the examination, especially if he is going to be interviewed or detained.

Asthma

Whenever a patient suffering from asthma requires medical assessment, the basic principles of the British Thoracic Society (BTS) Guidelines apply.

The following items need to be covered during the assessment.

- **Control of Symptoms** - Specific questions with regard to frequency of symptoms, presence of wheezing, breathlessness, coughing or chest tightness should be elicited as should diurnal and activity variations.

- **Current Medication** - The type of medication, delivery systems, and dosage should be obtained. The use of symptom led p.r.n. medication should be recorded. The ability to use the relevant delivery systems should be recorded.?

- **Examination** - As well as basic cardiorespiratory examination, the Peak Expiratory Flow Rate (PEF) should be measured. This should be compared with predicted rate and the best level recorded by the patient, if the latter knows it.

Once the above assessment has been completed, the decision with regard to fitness for detention can be made.

The medication schedule should be written out for the custody staff, as previously discussed above.

If well controlled, no change to the medication should be made. Occasionally the FME will see a detainee whose asthmatic symptoms are controlled by medication that is not in line with the BTS advice; on such occasions it may be appropriate to discuss the principles of treatment, and encourage the patient to seek a further consultation with his GP if released, or the Prison Medical Officer if remanded or detained. If the patient is remanded into police custody for more than a few days, it may be appropriate for such rationalisation of treatment to be undertaken by the police surgeon. No such treatment plan should be initiated without the police surgeon establishing either, that the prisoner will be under his/her care for long enough to stabilise the treatment, or appropriate communication with the responsible receiving physician, if relocation is planned.

If changes of medication are needed to establish control, the BTS stepwise approach is recommended – see text box overleaf. Any change in medication should be explained in detail to the detainee, reassurance being given and any fears addressed.

Management of chronic asthma

Step 1	Occasional use of relief bronchodilators	Inhaled, short acting β agonists prn. If needed >1/day ⇨ check technique, if ok ⇨ step 2
Step 2	Regular inhaled anti-inflammatory agents	Inhaled, short acting β agonists prn. + beclomethasone or budenoside 100-400 µg bd or try cromoglycate or nedocromil, but resort to steroids if no improvement is obtained with these.
Step 3	High dose inhaled	Inhaled, short acting β agonists prn. + steroids beclomethasone or budenoside 800-2000 µg daily via a large volume spacer or for those with difficulty with inhaled steroids a long acting β agonist or sustained release theophylline. Possibly try cromoglycate or nedocromil
Step 4	High dose inhaled steroids and regular bronchodilators	Inhaled, short acting β agonists prn. + beclomethasone or budenoside 800-2000 µg daily via a large volume spacer + a sequential therapeutic trial of one of:- • inhaled long acting β agonists • sustained release theophylline • inhaled ipatropium or oxitropium • long acting β agonist tablets • high-dose inhaled bronchodilators • cromoglycate or nedocromil
Step 5	Addition of regular oral steroids	Inhaled, short acting β agonists prn. + beclomethasone or budenoside 800-2000 µg daily via a large volume spacer + one or more long acting bronchodilators + regular prednisolone tabs in a single daily dose.

There are circumstances when rescue courses of oral steroids are required for the treatment of chronic asthma, but the detainee remains fit to be detained. These are:

• Symptoms and PEF get progressively worse by day
• Peak expiratory flow (PEF) falls below 60% of best
• Sleep is regularly disturbed by asthma
• There is diminishing response to inhaled bronchodilators

If these circumstances occur a dose of between 30-60 mg of prednisolone must be given in a single dose immediately and each morning until two days after control is re-established. A sufficient supply of oral steroids must, therefore, be prescribed.

If the detainee is leaving custody an appropriate written summary should be made available for the patient to take when property is returned, and/or transmitted to, for example, the patient's GP. Most custody suites have access to facsimile machines and many GP practices have them, so such information can be sent immediately.

As well as giving the oral steroids, adjustment to maintenance medication should be made in line with the stepwise approach.

Treatment of Acute Asthma[39]

(Advice following and "steps" reproduced with permission of BMA Specialist Journals)

1 Uncontrolled Asthma

    1.1 Assessment

        1.1.1 speech normal

        1.1.2 pulse <110/min

        1.1.3 respiration <25 breaths/ min

        1.1.4 PEF >50 % of predicted or best

    1.2 May be treated in custody with

        1.2.1 nebulised Salbutamol 5 mg **or**

        1.2.2 nebulised Terbutaline 10 mg **or**

        1.2.3 20-30 puffs of either drug via a large volume spacer

    1.3 Needs re-assessment in 15-30 minutes, if

        1.3.1 PEF remains 50-75%

            1.3.1.1 treat with oral steroids 30-60 mg prednisolone
            1.3.1.2 review after 4 hours

        1.3.2 if PEF >75% after 1.2

            1.3.2.1 step up usual treatment
            1.3.2.2 review after 4 hours

    1.4 Re-assessment after 4 hours

        1.4.1 PEF 50-75%

            1.4.1.1 nebulised Salbutamol 5 mg **or**
            1.4.1.2 nebulised Terbutaline 10 mg **or**
            1.4.1.3 20-30 puffs of either drug via a large volume spacer **and**
            1.4.1.4 start prednisolone 30-60 mg orally

1.5 Re-assessment after 15–30 minutes

    1.5.1 if no better refer to hospital

    1.5.2 if controlled with PEF >75% review 4 hours

    1.5.3 if then stable review ≤ 24 hours

1.6 Once started oral steroids should be continued until 2 days after control is re-established.

2 Acute Severe Asthma

2.1 Assessment

    2.1.1 can't complete sentences

    2.1.2 pulse ≥110/ min

    2.1.3 respiration ≥25 breaths /min

    2.1.4 PEF ≤50% of predicted or best

    2.1.5 but ≤33 % of predicted or best

2.2 If two or more of 2.1 are present admit to hospital

2.3 if one of 2.1 present treat as below **or admit to hospital**

    2.3.1 oxygen 40–60% *if available*

    2.3.2 nebulised Salbutamol 5 mg **or**

    2.3.3 nebulised Terbutaline 10 mg **or**

    2.3.4 20–30 puffs of either drug via a large volume spacer **and**

    2.3.5 start prednisolone 30–60 mg orally or 200 mg IV Hydrocortisone

2.4 Re-assessment after 15–30 minutes

    2.4.1 if no or little improvement **admit to hospital and whilst waiting with the patient for an ambulance**

        2.4.1.1 repeat initial inhaled treatment with the addition of nebulised Ipatropium 500 µg. **or**

        2.4.1.2 give subcutaneous Terbutaline **or**

        2.4.1.3 slow IV Aminophylline (**NB** not to be given if the patient is on oral theophyllines)

    2.4.2 if improved

        2.4.2.1 step up treatment **and**

        2.4.2.2 continue oral steroids

2.5 Re-assess in 4 hours

2.5.1 if stable

2.5.1.1 continue treatment and leave peak flow meter for self assessment every 4 hours

2.5.1.2 with the care instructions indicate a PEF below which further assessment needs to be made by a police surgeon.

3 Life Threatening Asthma

3.1 Assessment

3.1.1 silent chest

3.1.2 cyanosis

3.1.3 bradycardia or exhaustion

3.1.4 PEF <33% of best or predicted.

3.2 Arrange immediate hospital admission **and** treat with

3.2.1 Prednisolone 30-60 mg orally or 200 mg IV Hydrocortisone
3.2.2 Oxygen 40-60% *if available*

3.2.3 nebulised Salbutamol 5 mg **or**

3.2.4 nebulised Terbutaline 10 mg **or**

3.2.5 20-30 puffs of either drug via a large volume spacer **and**

3.2.6 Ipatropium 500 µgs via nebuliser **or**

3.2.7 give subcutaneous Terbutaline **or**

3.2.8 slow IV Aminophylline (**NB** not to be given if the patient is on oral Theophyllines)

3.3 Stay with the patient until the ambulance arrives.

HEAD INJURY AND ALTERED CONSCIOUSNESS

This may be the most difficult of all the medical problems in police cells. The first part of this section will concentrate on the head injury which is often found in association with alcohol misuse. It is extremely difficult to determine an objective degree of intoxication but this is discussed further in the following section headed "Intoxication".

A detailed history must be taken about how the injury occurred and at what time, i.e.:

- Was the patient knocked out and if so for how long?
- Can this be independently corroborated?
- Was there diplopia?
- Has he vomited since?
- Is the conscious level varying?

Remember the lucid interval in extradural haemorrhages

Remember the time lapse with subdural haemorrhages

The elderly and the neglected (alcoholics and malnourished) are more likely to get subdural haemorrhages.[40]

The examination will include a full CNS examination including examination of the fundi. Areas of contusion and lacerations will give an indication of the severity of the initial impact. Remember contra-coup injuries.

Major symptoms and signs for concern are:

- Pupil inequality
- Variable consciousness
- The fact that the person was knocked out
- Localising neurological signs
- Diplopia

Head injury warnings must be given to the officers and the police surgeon must return to reassess if he is worried. **TAKE NO RISKS - FATALITY AND MORBIDITY OCCUR TOO OFTEN.**

The head injured, intoxicated patient has been recognised for a considerable time as causing an assessment dilemma.

In the middle of the eighteenth century Sir Percival Pott was attributed with this

"A drayman, drunk and sleeping, fell from his dray.... He was brought to hospital senseless... the next day the man was so well and so perfectly the master of what sense he had, that I was inclined to believe that a great deal of last night's appearance was owing principally to the liquor".[41]

The discussion about the management of such patients has, as can be seen, been around for over 200 years.

For over a decade the management has been consolidated in various papers and advisory documents.

In 1986 the Royal College of Surgeons Commission on the provision of Surgical Services produced a *Report of the Working Party on Head Injuries*.

This report had a number of appendices giving tabulated advice and management aids.

Appendix III of this report was entitled *Guidelines for the Management of Patients with Recent Head Injury*. This guide listed the criteria for Skull X-ray, Hospital admission and Consultation with a Neurosurgical Unit.

The first two of these were thus:-

Criteria for Skull X-Ray after Recent Head Injury

Skull X-ray can be helpful but clinical judgement is necessary and the following criteria will be refined by further experience. The presence of one or more of the following indicates a need for skull X-ray in patients with a history of recent head injury.

1. Loss of consciousness or amnesia at any time
2. Neurological symptoms or signs
3. Cerebrospinal fluid or blood from nose or ear
4. Alcohol intoxication
5. Difficulty in assessing the patient

Note: Simple scalp laceration is not a criterion for skull X-ray.

Criteria for Hospital Admission after Recent Head Injury

The presence of one or more of the following

1. Confusion or any other depression of the level of consciousness at the time of examination
2. Skull fracture
3. Neurological signs or headache or vomiting
4. Difficulties in assessing the patient e.g. alcohol, the young, epilepsy
5. Other medical conditions - e.g. haemophilia
6. The patient's social conditions or lack of responsible adult/relative.

Note: a. Post-traumatic amnesia with full recovery is not an indication for admission

　　　b. Patients sent home should be given written instructions about possible complications and appropriate action.

The above guidelines had been based on over 15 years of research in the UK and the USA.

A later paper[42] examined retrospectively the application of these guidelines. The results of this research induced a recommendation from the authors to alter the criteria for referral for skull X-ray after recent head injury to:-

1. History of loss of consciousness or amnesia
2. Neurological signs or symptoms other than mild headache, dizziness or blurred vision.
3. CSF or blood from nose or ear.
4. Penetrating injury or scalp or periorbital bruising or swelling.
5. The elderly
6. If any of the above cannot be reliably excluded.

It can be seen that alcohol intoxication has been removed from this list. The reason for this being that the authors recommended that this combination needed **admission to hospital.**

It must be remembered that alcohol intoxication as well as predisposing to a risk of trauma[43] can also potentiate the symptoms of brain damage by causing a change in vascular tone and thrombocyte function, with a consequent risk of haemorrhage.[44] This same paper also drew attention to abuse of intoxicants other than alcohol as causing similar problems.

The paper by Mclaren *et al* referred to above[42] also suggested the alcohol intoxication group should include drug intoxicated patients. It also focused on the fact that intoxication was defined as abnormal behaviour and not just a history of alcohol consumption.

Criteria for Skull X-ray after Recent Head Injury	Criteria for Hospital Admission after Recent Head Injury
1. Loss of consciousness or amnesia at any time	1. Confusion or any other depression of the level of consciousness at the time of examination
2. Neurological symptoms or signs other than mild headache, dizziness or blurred vision.	2. Skull fracture
3. Cerebrospinal fluid or blood from nose or ear	3. Neurological signs or headache or vomiting
4. Penetrating injury or scalp or periorbital bruising or swelling.	4. Difficulties in assessing the patient e.g. the young, epilepsy
5. If any of the above cannot be reliably excluded	5. Other medical conditions - e.g. haemophilia
6. The elderly	6. The patient's social conditions or lack of responsible adult/relative.
	7. Alcohol or drug intoxication

Table 5.1

The question arises particularly in the custodial situation as to what constitutes a head injury.

Apocryphally most drunks in custody have some form of injury. The problem arises as to the differentiation between a cranial injury and a minor scalp or facial injury. Bleeding from the nose may only be due to damage to the nose and not the cranium or its contents. To some degree common sense must be used, but only after a detailed clinical appraisal of the situation such that the physician can show that any craniofacial injuries satisfy the conditions to **exclude** them from the guidelines which are summarised in Table 5.1 opposite.

Concussion is a transient and immediate loss of consciousness,[38] which may only last a few seconds, associated with a period of post traumatic amnesia[40] which may last considerably longer.

It should be remembered that about 3% of patients who have had concussion will have an intracranial haemorrhage. The risk is increased in the presence of a skull fracture.[38]

The assessment of other forms of altered consciousness is equally important. In the book by Plum & Posner[45] only 149 of 500 patients (none of course being in custody) who presented as Stupor or Coma of **Unknown Aetiology** were due to drug poisoning of one form or another.

If the patient is unconscious the decision is easier. But assessment of the degree of altered consciousness in the patient who is not comatose is more difficult.

Restricted neurological signs such as amnesia may reduce the total content of consciousness but are not normally regarded as an altered state of consciousness.[45] It can be vital for a police surgeon to accurately record the level of consciousness.

Labelling of the conscious level does not carry reliable agreed terminology for all levels, one of the problems being that altered consciousness does present as a continuum rather than stepped sequential conditions. Nevertheless it is not infrequent that an FME will be called upon to relate and justify the mental ability of a Solicitor's client, when the latter was a patient of that doctor, and just about to become a helper of the police with their inquiries.

So it is important that the physician determines semantics which are meaningful or at least consistent.

Various names have begun to have some definitive meaning: [45]

- Coma = Eyes closed, unresponsive even to noxious stimuli

- Stupor = Capable of being roused by vigorous and repeated stimuli, lapse back into "deep sleep" mode on ceasing of stimulus

- Obtundation = Means torpidity, reduced alertness and interest in environment, slow response to stimuli, and increased sleep

- Delirium = Floridly abnormal with disorientation, irritability, fear, sensory misperception and sometimes visual hallucination – may get lucid intervals.

- Clouding of = Reduced wakefulness **or** awareness, may have
  Consciousness irritability alternating with drowsiness. Attention reduced. Misjudgment of sensory perceptions, reduced rate and quality of cognition.

- Clouding of = As above but more advanced state with at least minor
  Consciousness disorientation to time and place, faulty memory, with
  with Confusion prominent drowsiness.

This degree of assessment becomes even more important in the case of examination for fitness to be interviewed which is dealt with in the next chapter.

Adequate examination and contemporaneous note keeping are mandatory.

It is vital to leave adequate instructions to the custody staff. Even though the discussion above has highlighted the diagnostic dilemma faced by trained physicians, there is still an expectation of producing simple guidelines for a lay person to follow in regard to the risk for late complications of head injury (See Note b. of the original working party on page 63). The typical instructions given when a patient is discharged from casualty is all one can expect a police officer to carry out. It is not appropriate to ask a custody officer to carry out sequential 15 minute Glasgow Coma Scores.

Having clinically assessed a patient as not needing referral to hospital then simple written instructions on the lines shown in Table 5.2 should be given to the custody staff or the patient if the latter is being released from custody.

Head Injury Instructions For Custody Officers
If a detainee after a head injury:-

1.   Becomes unconscious
    2.   Becomes increasingly sleepy
    3.   Complains of increasingly severe headache
    4.   Complains of blurred or double vision
    5.   Vomits
    6.   Has a fit

The medical officer must be contacted. If immediate response from the physician is not obtained the detainee must be taken to the nearest Accident & Emergency department at once.

Table 5.2

INTOXICATION AND SUBSTANCE ABUSE

The booklet *Guidelines for the Clinical Management of Substance Misuse Detainees in Police Custody* produced by the Department of Health, Scottish Office Home & Health Department and Welsh Office and available from HMSO should be mandatory reading for all police surgeons.

General Points

Substance abuse is common. In some areas it appears that illicit drugs have supplanted alcohol as the commonest intoxicants seen in detainees.

The problem is a huge one to society and this is amply illustrated in The White Paper *Tackling Drugs Together, 1995-1998.*

The approach to the assessment of the intoxicated patient should be the same whatever substance is suspected, and should include a comprehensive physical examination and mental state assessment. This takes on an added importance when it may be offered by a defendant that he did not have the mens rea for a particular offence. This has been highlighted recently in a Law Commission report.[46]

It may become crucial for a proper assessment of intoxication vs other causes of consciousness disturbance to have been made so that appropriate opinion may be drawn from the contemporaneous medical documents.

The FME has a unique opportunity to intervene in a drug user's career at a time of crisis when they may be receptive to new ideas and advice. Greater Manchester Police have a policy of disseminating information about the Specialist Drug Services to all detainees, but even where this service is provided it does no harm to induce the patient to think about seeking treatment, or at least to consider risk minimisation practises.

The forensic clinician must have a good working knowledge of the following in order to fulfill his/her responsibilities to the substance misuser:-

1. The signs of intoxication with alcohol and medical or psychiatric conditions which may mimic them.

2. The signs of intoxication with the common drugs of abuse:
    2.1 both illegal, e.g. heroin, cocaine, amphetamines, cannabis, LSD
    2.2 prescribed, e.g. benzodiazepine, cyclizine
    2.3 legal OCPs[g], e.g. Aztec Black Resin

and the medical conditions which mimic these.

---

g. Over the counter products from some shops, not usually from high street shops or pharmacies.

It must be remembered that drugs are often taken in combination, by varying routes and in comparatively high doses.

3. The stigmata of chronic drug and alcohol misuse.

4. The physical complications of drug and alcohol misuse.

5. The features of withdrawal states, and the appropriate treatment.

6. A good working knowledge of local patterns of drug misuse and treatment options.

That substance misuse is a potent risk factor for suicide has been recognised for a considerable time, with relation to alcohol[47] and to drugs.[48] High dose stimulant users, especially cocaine and amphetamine, may develop a withdrawal depressive state within the first 7-10 days of abstinence, which of course can carry a concomitant suicidal risk.

In addition many drug misusers have depression and/or anxiety, and some represent a sub-group with a vulnerable personality, though it is unclear exactly how much of the clinical illness may pre-date the substance misuse.[49]

Many substance abusers are protected from the reality of the unacceptable aspects of their lives by the drug induced state, and withdrawal may precipitate them back into that reality.

Serious physical disease may co-exist with drug abuse, and may need urgent intervention.

Although alcohol and drug misuse, in themselves, are specifically excluded from the terms of the Mental Health Act 1983 (MHA)[50] as reasons for compulsory admission to hospital, if a recognised mental illness is present which satisfies the criteria of the MHA with regard to formal admission, then the act can be applied even if the mental illness is considered to be as a consequence of the substance misuse.

DEALING WITH THE SUBSTANCE MISUSER

The substance abuser demands the same standard of care, treatment and respect as does any patient. The advice on consent and section should be read (Chapters 2 & 3).

Medication brought into custody, if identifiable as a properly dispensed medication, forms part of the detainee's property and if unused should be returned to him on release. This caveat also applies to licitly provided needles and syringes.

The FME must use his/her clinical skills to assess

- The degree of intoxication
- What substances are involved
- Is the patient habituated to the substances
- Has an overdose been taken
- Are there any signs or symptoms of withdrawal
- Is there any other disease process or injury present (e.g. epilepsy, head injury *v.s.*)
- Is he fit to detain
- Is review needed and if so when
- What treatment, if any, is needed

If the degree of intoxication leads to a degree of clouding of consciousness, but after due consideration the FME has decided that this state is not a hazard, it must be decided whether regular rousing is appropriate. This may depend on many factors and the degree of intoxication per se is one of them.

Some recent work has drawn attention to the importance and ease[51] of assessing alcohol in custody and the incidence, prevalence and ease of use of a breath analysis device in custody.[52] Hand held devices are ideal, but may be considered expensive. It may be possible to use the Lion Intoximeter (or Camic device) to breathalyse the detainee to estimate the blood alcohol level (multiply the breathalyser reading by a factor of 2.3 $\simeq$ blood alcohol). Such usage would depend on the procedural availability of such devices and the consciousness and co-operation of the detainee.

Finally, if the detainee is to be left in custody, the FME must determine an appropriate time for clinical re-assessment, if such is needed. This information should be written along with the care and advice notes left for the custody staff.

If referral to hospital is required, standard local conventions as regard to such arrangements should be honoured. The FME is in a unique position, however, and once a sensible decision has been made to refer for assessment or admission, that decision should not be responsive to pressure to change.

Whatever treatment schedule is decided, clear written instructions must be given to the custody staff (see page 50). The police surgeon should not assume that a police officer is familiar with all the complications that may ensue in the intoxicated patient. Examples of this are the risk of inhaled vomit or fits. If the prisoner is soundly asleep (the dilemmas often present at night), the officers should be instructed to put him in the recovery position. It may be appropriate, for caution, to have the detainee roused regularly. He must be roused to such an extent that he performs simple movements and responds appropriately to commands. Any "change for the worse" in his condition must be notified to the Police Surgeon. In particular, this means increasing drowsiness, lack of response, severe headache and persistent vomiting. There have been suggestions that rousing every 15 minutes should be used. The current Codes of Practice (PACE) carry a new para-

PRINCIPLES OF FORENSIC MEDICINE

graph in Code C. This paragraph, 8.10 on page 46, actually states that " A person who is drunk shall be roused and spoken to on each visit. [see *Note 8A*]". *Note 8A states " Whenever possible juveniles and other people at risk should be visited more frequently"*. However this procedure and rousing every 15 minutes does seem questionable in general medical terms. If the doctor is concerned enough to have such frequent rousing then the surgeon should remain on the premises until the clinical appraisal allows a more appropriate decision to be made, or until admission is arranged, if that is the disposal decided upon. There appears to be no medical condition which could safely be left in the hands of observing police officers, and which could deteriorate at a rate for which 15 minute observations would allow appropriate intervention to take place, yet avoid calamity in the interval. 30 minute observations seem reasonable.

In addition to the observational instructions and criteria the FME has a duty to advise the custody staff about dangers to others. This may relate to specific problems such as the build up of volatile substances in small spaces, in which solvent abusers are contained and to more general policies regarding infection risk.

The concept of designating infection risk by known status such as HIV +ve has been shown to be invalid,[53] and therefore it is good practice for the treatment and handling of all detainees to follow sound Occupational Health guidelines. Such guidelines will be available from the Occupational Health Service of the Force.

Acute intoxication with stimulants may present with hyper-excitability, and the cessation of this should be marked with increased vigilance.

No intoxicated detainee with reduced level of consciousness should be left in custody without at least one assessment of a blood sugar. It should not be forgotten that hypoglycaemia may cause confusion and/or abnormal behaviour long before unconsciousness.

Hypoglycaemia, caused by primary underproduction of glucose, in the intoxicated patient, is due to the effect alcohol has on hepatic gluconeogenesis.[38] Though this will only occur when the patient has suffered a period of fasting which has depleted liver glycogen stores, such a presentation is not unlikely in the patient subgroup seen in custody. Assuming a hypoglycaemic coma to be the stuporous sleep of the drunkard is unacceptable.

The malnourished high dose stimulant user may also run into hypoglycaemic problems after a violent arrest.

Substitution treatment for the illicit drug user is a constant cause of problems for the FME.

The classical case is that of opioid abuse. Many detainees are also on legally prescribed opioids, but experience has shown that many of these are also still using illicit forms of the drug. The advice given in general in the booklet referred to at the start of this section (see page 67) should be strongly considered with regard to the whole range of drugs.

The FME should ask about prescribed medication, and look into confirmation of this if possible. If properly prescribed the police surgeon should consider continuing the medication. Blanket bans on the prescribing of particular drugs are untenable and unethical. However each case must be judged on its own merits.

The clinical well-being of the patient is the primary concern. However many detention areas provide a unique problem for the physician. This problem particularly applies to remand prisoners. In these circumstances the FME may have a large number of addicts, sometimes sharing a cell with one or two others and having a fair amount of free association with others in the block. The potential within this closed captive community for manipulation and social disharmony is enormous. The FME must carefully consider the treatment programmes on firm clinical assessment alone of each individual. A high degree of communication with the patients is necessary to maintain any form of doctor/patient relationship or trust. Firmness and consistency are, however, absolutely imperative.

Where the decision is taken to discontinue a prescribed drug, not only should that be recorded in the FME's notes but also explained to the patient.

Though a controlled drug subject to the Misuse of Drugs Act 1971 cannot be administered by a police officer, such a drug may be self administered under the personal supervision of a police surgeon.

This rule is now embodied in the new Codes (of PACE) which states that this personal supervision will have been satisfied if the custody officer consults the police surgeon. The particular section[54] indicates that this may be done by telephone.

Though it may be appropriate for a police surgeon to ratify, by telephone, the continuation of identifiable simple drugs, such as mild analgesics or a partially completed course of antibiotics, it is not appropriate for opioids to be given without a full clinical assessment. Once the assessment has been made, there is no need for the police surgeon to be present when the patient takes the medication, and it would be good practice to provide a course of the drug chosen for the time the detainee is likely to be in custody, though weekly review would be appropriate.

If the doctor is prescribing a controlled drug (CD)[h] the prescription must be a private one (see page 52) and the handwriting and format requirements must also be observed.

If a CD is to be prescribed then methadone is the drug of choice. It should be used in liquid form (but see next chapter on Fitness for Interview) and even though, because of its long half life it may be given as a single daily dose, twice daily administration is often preferred by the patient and, particularly where a comparatively large dose is needed, is often safer.

---

h. In this text "Controlled Drug" refers to those preparations which are subject to The Misuse of Drugs (Notification of and Supply to Addicts) Regulations 1973 (see page 25).

If the FME decides not to prescribe a CD, then other appropriate symptomatic treatment should be considered. Dihydrocodeine is a suitable alternative. In theory the withdrawal of opioids can cause a noradrenergic crisis and could lead to severe cardiovascular problems. The patient should be examined with this complication in mind. The booklet mentioned at the beginning of this chapter (see page 49) contains an overview of the treatment and is recommended reading.

If the detainee is pregnant, sudden withdrawal of opiates may be life threatening to the fetus in the first trimester and may cause premature labour and stillbirth later. In such circumstances methadone substitution or continuation is mandatory. If substitution is needed this should be instituted in hospital. A woman may claim she is in the early stages of pregnancy. Under these circumstances a pregnancy test using one of the various testing kits will assist the doctor in his/her therapeutic decision. It is worthwhile carrying one of these kits in the medical bag. If there is any doubt about the stability of the pregnant opioid addict then admission is the best policy.

The fact that a patient is for example, a heroin addict, does not exclude them from any concommittant disease, and all aspects of their health should be dealt with.

Complications of the drug abuse, eg an injection site abscess, which needs treatment, should be dealt with.

The police surgeon is reminded about the statutary duties with regard to notification covered in Chapter 3.

Benzodiazepine dependence is common both in isolation and together with other drugs.

If the patient gives a history indicating such dependence then benzodiazepines must not be stopped abruptly as this may lead to convulsions, or occasionally acute psychosis. Cover of sudden benzodiazepine withdrawal may be treated with carbamazepine, though until more work has been done on this, it is not recommended in custody.

Substance abusers may have developed tolerance to huge doses of benzodiazepines, which may be taken by various routes. They may in addition abuse alcohol.

It is good practice to convert all the benzodiazepines used to a long-acting equivalent such as diazepam or chlordiazepoxide and to prescribe this in three or four daily doses. Unless there is the complication of added acute alcohol withdrawal then a maximum dose of 80 mg of diazepam in 24 hours should not be exceeded. Conversion equivalents of the common benzodiazepines are shown in Table 5.3.

On occasions detainees may be so intoxicated and violent (usually after taking high doses of stimulants, eg crack, cocaine or amphetamines, or hallucinogenics) that they require restraint in order to prevent their harming others or them-

Approximate equivalent doses to 5 mg diazepam [37]	
Chlordiazepoxide	15 mg
Loprazolam	0.5-1mg
Lorazepam	0.5 mg
Lormetazepam	0.5-1mg
Nitrazepam	5 mg
Oxazepam	15 mg
Temazepam	10 mg

Table 5.3

selves. It should be borne in mind that "hog-tying" (wrists and ankles bound and then tied to each other behind the back) has been associated with a number of deaths in the USA.[55,56] If that degree of restraint is necessary, the limbs should be fastened in front of the body, for as short a time as possible, and the prisoner left under permanent observation until appropriate clinical disposal or treatment has been arranged. Plasticuffs should be used, not ridgid linked cuffs.

INTIMATE SEARCHES

An "Intimate Search" arises under section 55 of PACE and is defined further under Annex A of paragraph 4.1 of section C of the Codes of Practice. This has recently been modified by s59 of the Criminal Justice and Public Order Act 1994.

Such a search is defined as a "physical examination of a person's body orifices other than the mouth."

The statutory criteria needing to be met are succinctly documented in the new Codes and will not be reproduced here, as a copy of the Codes should always be available.

An intimate search should not be made lightly by a police surgeon. The ethic of infringing an individual's rights by enforced search was highlighted by BMA policy in 1988[57] thus:-

"That this meeting believes that no medical practitioner should take part in an intimate body search of a subject without that subject's consent". Attention was drawn to this again in the publication *Health Care of Detainees in Police Stations*.

Though the FME may be protected from criminal charges if such a non-consensual examination is done, the crux of the matter is the ethic of such a procedure, including the aspects of apparent consent under duress or coercion. The history of the physician's ethic in this has been re-iterated strongly thus:-

The Hippocratic Oath

> "...I will prescibe regimen for the good of my patients according to my ability and my judgement and never do harm to anyone...."

International Code of Medical Ethics

> "...ANY ACT OR ADVICE which could weaken physical or mental resistence of a human being may be used only in his interest..."

Declaration of Tokyo, 1975

> "1. The doctor shall not countenannce, condone or participate in the practice of torture or other forms of cruel, inhuman or degrading procedures, whatever the offence of which the victim of such procedures is suspected, accused or guilty...."

A digital examination of such as the vagina or anus, without consent, has to be considered to be a degrading procedure. If connected with drug "packing" there is also the risk of rupture of the package with consequent absorption of the contents. The police surgeon must carefully consider all aspects of the case in great detail, including the potential risk to others in society, and alternative methods which may be available to achieve the discovery of drugs or an article which may cause injury to the potential examinee or others, before making a decision. A simple blanket decision to say "no" could be deemed to be an abrogation of social duty, if lacking reasoned argument to back it up, just as much as an automatic agreement to perform these examinations could break faith with a basic tenet of medical ethic. There should be no coercion on the potential examinee **nor** on the doctor to partake in any such examination.

The doctor should be familiar with the amended BMA policy document which also states "...except on very rare occasions..an intimate search should not be carried out without the subject's consent". The reference between "occasions" and "an intimate" in the above extract refers to a search with regard to an object which could cause physical injury. The document goes on to indicate that policy will not support a doctor examining without consent for an object which will harm the subject himself, though where others may be at risk it is conceded that it may be necessary to carry out the search, but that the doctor should be aware of BMA policy and justify his/her actions. Under this section the police can carry out the search themselves.

The BMA policy document should be read in full.

6

FITNESS TO BE INTERVIEWED

FITNESS TO
BE INTERVIEWED

This area of the police surgeons work has steadily grown in the last few years from an embryo to a potential monster.

There has been no formal training on the subject, the expectations placed upon FMEs vary depending on the particular interest, slant and responsibility of the lay professional viewing the doctor, and it is unclear exactly what is the responsibility of the police surgeon.

It appears that this whole area of work stemmed from the original Codes of Practice constituting **s 66** of the Police and Criminal Evidence Act 1984 (PACE).

In this chapter and Chapter 11 on Mental Health when referring to the codes of practice in general, the PACE codes will be referred to as Codes (PACE) and the Codes of Practice of the Mental Health Act 1983 will be referred to as Codes (MHA).

In paragraph 12.3 of Code C of PACE it states

"No person who is unfit through drink or drugs to the extent that he is unable to appreciate the significance of questions put to him and his answers may be questioned about an alleged offence in that condition except in accordance with Annex C. [See *Note 12C*]"

Annex C is still extant and is discussed on page 86.

Note 12B states

" The police surgeon can give advice about whether or not a person is fit to be interviewed in accordance with paragraph 12.3 above".

There is no mention of the police surgeon being involved with regard to fitness for interview in any other condition including mental health disorders.

The only apparent change between the original Codes (PACE) and the current edition which became effective on 10 April 1995 is that *Note 12C* had become *Note 12B* on publication of the second draft of the Codes (PACE) and remains so.

There is mention of calling the police surgeon, and immediately so, if a person brought to the police station appears to be suffering from a mental illness or is incoherent except through drunkenness alone,[58] but there is no mention of involvement with fitness for interview.

However it is apocryphally stated that FMEs are involved in fitness to be interviewed for many detainees suffering from a legion of conditions.

There is no claim in this text that such a use of forensic clinicians is improper, but it is an area which had not been specifically researched with a goal of producing set parameters for such an assessment.

As there are no set protocols to assess fitness for interview, this rests with the clinical judgement of the forensic clinician in attendance.

It is interesting that the *Victoria Police Forensic Medical Officers Manual*, published in 1992 written and compiled by Drs David Wells, Edward Ogden, Simon Young and Faika Jappie, adopted a similar approach to this in their advice for fitness to interview.

That Manual states:

"You do not have to make a definitive diagnosis. You simply need to establish:-

1. Is (s)he mentally alert and orientated to answer questions?
2. Is (s)he physically well enough to answer questions?"

Other work which will be mentioned may suggest that more needs to be done than answering the simple questions above.

This chapter will explore this area and, for convenience only, the subject has been split into the following headings:

General Aspects
Clinical Assessment of Interviewee
Responsibilities of Forensic Clinician

GENERAL ASPECTS

There has been much publicity and, now, not inconsiderable work on false confessions.

Though the FME cannot audit interrogation techniques, they can do their best to apply their clinical skills to identify vulnerable patients.

It must be remembered that not everyone interviewed is in detention. Not everyone interviewed is a suspect. A police surgeon may come across a situation where they are asked to assess an individual who is a complainant or a non participating witness to the alleged events.

The assessment for fitness to be interviewed could be considered to be threefold. Firstly that an interview, which may be verbally rigorous, does no harm. Secondly that the interviewee is fit such that they are capable of recall and recounting the "facts". Lastly, that they are not so vulnerable that they are unduly open to suggestibility. It should be remembered that most people are suggestible to a certain extent

Once the clinician is satisfied that the patient is not at risk of either of the first two of these aspects, it should be remembered that the patient's opinion on this subject matters. As a point of principle the detainee should always be asked if they have any objection or comment to make on the subject of interview. Many will wish to be interviewed as soon as possible, in order (or in hope) that they will then be released to go about their daily business. The third aspect will be seen to evolve as the chapter progresses.

Even though much of the text will refer to a "detainee" from a point of simplicity, the information and opinion that follows applies equally to any interviewee, whether they be a suspect or not, except of course to any specifics about custodial care.

It has already been alluded to that no satisfactory publication exists to help the forensic clinician in this specific task. In earlier chapters (1 & 4) mention has been made of the importance of full contemporaneous notes. The situation of fitness for interview is a classic example of the importance of complete and comprehensive records. If the FME has made a satisfactory assessment, recorded the clinical findings in detail and given appropriate opinion, then no problem should later ensue in court.

Consent should be sought and considered a forensic examination; this is covered in Chapter 2 under Fitness for Interview.

CLINICAL ASSESSMENT OF INTERVIEWEE

The previous chapter on Fitness to be Detained should be read.

Physical illness

Any detainee who is suffering from a specific physical illness should be stable before interview takes place. It is difficult to be specific. For example the hypertensive does not have to be normotensive, only preferably so. Some hypertensive patients are stable at a theoretically hypertensive level. It behoves the clinician to establish, if possible, the "normal" state for that patient, if a higher blood pressure reading than expected is obtained. This, of course, can be a difficult or even impossible task in the middle of the night, in which case the clinical judgement of the FME must be exercised. A similar approach can also be taken towards other conditions such as diabetes mellitus. In the latter case no clinical appraisal should be considered complete without a blood sugar estimation.

If a patient is on medication then the treatment protocol should be ratified and written up on whatever is the accepted format for care instructions for detainees (see Appendix 3c for the example of the Greater Manchester Police form).

The detainee who is injured or suffering from a musculoskeletal disorder needs assessing and any appropriate analgesia given. If serious injury is considered they should have that condition assessed and treated before interview. *The British National Formulary* (BNF) describes both Aspirin and Paracetamol as particularly useful for musculoskeletal pain and pyrexia. The former can be used (if not contra-indicated in the individual) where anti-inflammatory action is required. The BNF points out that any combined analgesic, containing an opioid, has no substantiated benefit over the simple drug, if the dose is low, and carries all the side effects of the opioid if containing a higher dose.

Visceral pain is however more responsive to opioid analgesics.

Care must be taken not to give an opioid analgesia in a dose which may cause drowsiness, during the interview, in a patient unused to strong drugs.

In police surgeon practice the above example infrequently presents. The specific case of drug addicts is dealt with below.

Examination

The examination should include:-

1. A full medical history including family, social, and past medical/surgery/ (obstetric) histories.
2. Medication details including any alcohol or illicit drugs used.

   2.1 For illicit drugs it is of help to use the regional data base forms as part of the medical record (see Chapter 3 Section and Appendices 3a & b).

   2.2 It is worthwhile remembering the availability of legal "herbal" highs.

   2.3 The history should include habitual use as well as intake in the last 24 hours.
3. Nutrition

   3.1 General condition, and

   3.2 Food intake - when and what?
4. Full clinical examination with particular reference to stigmata of drug abuse and/or withdrawal.

   4.1 Does the patient normally wear spectacles (or contact lenses)?, or

   4.2 Have a hearing deficit?
   (important if going to be interviewed or asked to sign anything).
5. The CNS examination should include.

   5.1 Locomotor function.

   5.2 Co-ordination.

   5.3 Temporo-spatial orientation.

5.4 Cognitive function

5.5 Short memory recall

The standard questions of   Where are you?
                            What day is it?
                            What time is it?
                            Why are you here?
                            Who are you?
                                (i.e. what is your name, where do you live etc?)
                            Who is that?
                                (e.g. identification of police officer, doctor,
                                another prisoner)

referred to by Myles Clarke[59] as Kipling's 'five men', who, where, when, what and how, can often be sufficient to establish orientation in space and time

The classic questions of naming the Prime Minister, and/or a recent news item, remembering a name and address given to him a few minutes before, and taking serial 7's from 100 are all suitable tests for cognition.

The depth of the assessment is important. A paper by Gudjonsson[60] develops the subject based on a case where he gave evidence as an expert. The accused had been declared fit for interview by an FME and a consultant psychiatrist and was attended by an approved social worker as the appropriate adult (see below). After expert evidence by Gudjonsson the interview statements were declared as being inadmissable by the judge. There was no question of improper behaviour by the police in interview technique, but it was apparent that the medical assessment had not considered all three aspects as mentioned above under the section on **General Aspects** but had only considered the first of these. The importance in this case was the assessment of the reliability of the patient.

Some cautionary notes should be remembered at this stage.

Those without employment or ordered social life, a not unusual finding in the patients in custody, may often have little idea of the day of the week, just as some police surgeons lose track of the day when on two weeks, leave.

Though no research has been discovered relating to this, it appears that a large proportion of examinees under the age of 35 appear to have difficulty with the serial 7 subtraction even with otherwise apparent normal cognition. Rather than assume that a poor performance of this test demonstrates a lack of higher mental functions, the assessment should be viewed as a whole or a simpler test such as taking away progressive 3's or 4's should be attempted. It has been apocryphally mentioned that this age group represents a threshold of the population who were still at school when the market was flooded with electronic pocket calculators, which co-incided with the demise of learning "times tables etc".

Psychiatric problems

Any indication of depression, thought disorder, delusions or abnormal behaviour should be examined more deeply.

Depression, other than mild depression, may be accompanied by psycho-motor retardation, and poor memory. Anxiety and agitation can co-exist. A careful assessment must be made before declaring any apparently depressed patient fit for interview.

Anxiety itself can be induced in the innocent by interrogation[61] and should not therefore be taken as an obstruction for interview. The degree of anxiety, however, should be assessed and discussed with the patient. Such a discussion itself may resolve much of the anxiety without further interference. Many of the unpleasant symptoms of anxiety may be controlled by a small dose of β blockade which should not affect cognitive function.

Patients with active severe disease such as mania, psychosis, schizophrenia-like disorders will not be fit for interview (see Chapter 11 for a discussion of mental health).

Alcohol

The alcoholic patient should be assessed as with any patient. The mere label of alcoholism does not bar the patient from interview.

Alcohol intoxication is another matter.

It has been suggested that the level set by the Road Traffic Acts of 80 mg of alcohol per 100 ml (%) of blood should be a level, above which, a patient is unfit for interview.[59] This opinion, in an otherwise excellent paper, appears to have no sound basis.

There has been much research on drinking and driving and there appears to be no doubt that the risk of accident at the current legal UK limit is twice that of the alcohol free driver.[62] At the same level the younger driver has a five fold increased risk of accident. This itself shows a variation in individual response. Young people, due to a greater susceptibility to alcohol, less driving experience, social behaviour patterns, or a combination of any of these are more affected. To set an arbitrary limit of a Blood Alcohol Concentration (BAC) of 80 mg % cannot be supported. As a BAC of about 1500 mg % has been survived[63] it can be seen that not only can massive tolerance develop but that in such a case even with a twofold increase[i] in the liver's ability to metabolise alcohol, it would be two days before such an individual could be interviewed. This presentation sets an artificial argument which is extreme, particularly as the patient would likely be in hospital, but it is used to illustrate the point that an artificially set level of

---

i. i.e. eliminating the ethanol from the blood at about 30mgs % /hour.

BAC is not an adequate yardstick. It may help to measure the BAC and this can be done with the breath devices in the police station, if such is acceptable within the Force Orders or by a hand held breath alcohol measurement device. Such a reading would be only one facet of a comprehensive clinical evaluation.

It has recently been suggested by Robertson *et al*[64] that the idea suggested by Clarke above "has considerable merit", "and if no medical or drug related complications are suspected, there is no reason why doctors need be involved in the procedure as the police are perfectly capable of using the instrument themselves." Though the caveat of medical and drug problems is mentioned in the article, the suggestion itself must rely on the police officer concerned diagnosing the absence of clinical abnormality. Such would not be a pathway of safety for the patient. In his article, cited above, Clarke does mention that even when the BAC has dropped to the acceptable limit, clinical re-assessment should be undertaken.

The decision on fitness for interview should be made on a clinical assessment.

Drug addiction

The drug addict poses specific problems.

Guidance does now exist with regard to this problem in the form of the booklet *Guidelines for the Clinical Management of Substance Misuse Detainees in Police Custody.*

This publication is issued by the
  Department of Health
  Scottish Office Home and Health Department
  Welsh Office

This became available in 1994 and it is meant to be complementary to *Drug Misuse and Dependence - Guidelines on Clinical Management*

This booklet, available since 1991 from HMSO, is published by the same government offices.

The later supplement had significant input from the Association of Police Surgeons (APS) in the persons of the then President of the APS, Dr Ralph Lawrence, Dr Peter Green and Dr Margaret Stark.

Forensic Clinicians should be familiar with the content of both booklets.

With regard to fitness to interview, two questions will undoubtedly arise in connection with the addict:

1. was the withdrawal complex severe enough to cause a physical and mental debility sufficient to invalidate the recall of the witness or to result in a distress sufficient to lead to false confessions?

2. did the administration of the dependency substance adversely affect the cognitive function of the interviewee?

In his book[61] Gudjonsson drew attention to the lack of research in the area of the effect of drug and alcohol withdrawal on accuracy and completeness of testimony. He cited one paper,[65] but also noted a serious methodological problem with it, that concluded there was no significant difference in suggestibility between addicts and non-addicts. That was in 1992. Work done since then has possibly supported that finding. Gudjonsson *et al*[66] found that the "consumption of alcohol or illicit drugs up to 24 hours prior to arrest did not load saliently on any of the factors". The "factors" in this research were mental health, memory and suggestibility, previous criminality and literacy and IQ. One reason given as to why this should be so was that substance abuse shortly prior to arrest may have had relatively little effect on the subjects mental state. Such a view is supported by another paper.[67]

The research mentioned above[66] took up to one hour to assess each detainee. Police surgeons have neither the time nor the psychological skills to do such an assessment, but the work would suggest that a comprehensive and detailed examination by the physician is appropriate.

The decision on fitness for interview should be made on a clinical assessment.

If an opioid addict is showing significant signs of withdrawal, including those signs which are difficult to mimic, such as gooseflesh, tachycardia, increased bowel sounds, pupillary dilatation, then he is unlikely to be fit for interview without therapy. It may be that the detainee will be released after interview, and the physician has a responsibility to the patient to expedite the interview, rather than allow him to languish in custody for an unreasonable time, until his symptoms allow him to be interrogated.[j] Such an end may be reached by the administration of a small dose of methadone, and physeptone tablets are easily carried in the medical bag for this purpose. However the treatment decision is one that can only be made by the physician in attendance and there are other treatment options available. The guidelines referred to at the beginning of this section carry good advice about withdrawal therapy.

The other question that arises relates to the window of opportunity for completing an interview.

If the FME declares a detainee to be fit for interview, that declaration is valid at the time it was written, presuming pen was put to paper immediately at the end of the examination. The forensic clinician must make it clear that such is the case. In the vast majority of detainees the examination findings should hold fast for 3-4 hours (as long as a new event does not intervene). If the interview is delayed for any reason beyond that time scale then the interviewee will need to be re-assessed.

If the detainee is declared not fit for interview, and interview will be required at

---

j. "interview" and "interrogate" are considered to have exactly the same meaning in this text.

some stage, then the police surgeon should indicate a time when the patient can be re-assessed clinically. There may be some cases, such as the detainee, late at night, with a degree of intoxication, and fatigue, who would be better left to sleep overnight, in which case the FME may wish to indicate the time that interview could take place without re-assessment. It is recommended that this should only occur with a known individual, such that no other mental problems might be masked by the transient symptoms and signs.

This advice is included in the section devoted to the substance abuser, but the concept equally applies to any circumstance.

RESPONSIBILITIES OF THE FORENSIC CLINICIAN

Appropriate adult

The appropriate adult (AA) was born fully grown but seemingly immature with PACE in 1984. The role appears to be increasing. This increase seems to be a consequence of heightened awareness of the need for an AA rather than a change in the dimensions of their responsibilities.

The AA is recommended for

> juveniles (Codes (PACE) C 1.7 (a))
> a person who is mentally disordered or mentally handicapped
> (Codes (PACE) C 1.7 (b))

Sections 1.4 and 1.5 of the Codes (PACE), immediately preceding the above sections, indicate that if the custody officer is suspicious or is informed in good faith that either apply, then the detainee shall be treated as though the category did apply.

The responsibility to call an AA lies with the custody officer.

It should be made clear, however, in any instructions given to the custody officer by the FME, whether he/she believes an AA should be involved. It may be all too easy for a busy custody officer to assume that when a detainee has been passed fit for interview by a police surgeon, then, for example, significant mental disorder does not exist, unless the doctor has so indicated.

The research by Nemitz and Bean[68] appears to indicate that this reliance on the police surgeon is an active if informal reality. In this paper the authors have highlighted an important area which could be fraught with misunderstanding.

The recently re-designed Fitness to be Detained form (Form 717) of Greater Manchester Police, illustrated in Appendix 3c, has areas which the police surgeon can fill in easily by deletion of alternatives, such that specific opinion is expressed.

The FME should express an opinion one way or another.

Any doubt should always be expressed to favour the detainee with the benefit of that doubt and for an AA to be recommended.

The responsibilities of an AA are laid down in the Codes (PACE) in **C** paragraph 11.16. There it is clearly stated that the AA is not just there as an observer but should also

1

1.1 Advise the person being questioned

1.2 Observe whether or not the interview is being conducted properly and fairly

2 Facilitate communication with the person being interviewed.

In the case of a juvenile the parent can act as the AA. What has not been made clear is the assessment of the competency of the AA. It is possible that the most caring parent may not make the best AA for the offspring for a number of reasons.

It is important that the forensic clinician is aware of the responsibilities of mental health in the custodial situation and further aspects of such work is covered in Chapter 11.

Annex C

Annex C of the Codes C(PACE) is present to avoid delay in gaining necessary information which otherwise is

"likely

(a) to lead to interference with or harm to evidence connected with an offence or interference with or physical harm to other people;"[69]

This annex allows vulnerable subjects to undergo urgent interviews, overriding the safeguards designed to protect them. The urgent interview must end as soon as the information is available which will avert the risk mentioned above.

The FME should be aware of this as clinical assessment for fitness to be interviewed may be requested after the urgent interview has taken place.

Remember

The decision on fitness for interview should be made on a clinical assessment.

QUICK REFERENCE

- Is the patient medically fit to be interviewed?

- Is the patient a juvenile (ie under 17 years)?
  > Recommend an Appropriate Adult
  > (can be a parent)

- Is the patient mentally disordered or mentally handicapped?
  > Recommend an Appropriate Adult

- Has the patient any other disabilities, eg Hearing or visual impairment?
  > Draw this to the attention of the custody officer

- Decide on re-assessement time (if appropriate)?

7

EXAMINATION IN CASES OF ASSAULT

EXAMINATION IN CASES OF ASSAULT

The examination of a patient in the case of an alleged assault should follow the same pattern whether the examinee is the complainant or accused.

Standard medical history taking techniques should be involved

- Introduction
- Consent
- History
- Examination
- Investigation
- Diagnosis

The "Diagnosis" in the forensic context, of course, as has been alluded to in other chapters, is a formulation of opinion about causation.

INTRODUCTION

The FME should introduce him/herself to the patient explaining

1. The purpose of the examination
2. The procedure to be adopted
3. The investigations needed to be done (if any)

CONSENT

Consent should then be taken, including explicit parameters regarding disclosure, investigation and photography etc. Chapter 2 on Consent should be read.

HISTORY

The history of the alleged events insofar as that history has a direct bearing on the clinical appraisal should be taken.

Account must also be taken of factors which may affect such an appraisal. This would include any intoxicants, or other drugs, past medical and surgical history, any medication being taken, and any social history which may reflect on the condition of the patient, such as homelessness and having lived "rough". Any other recent physical confrontation, of any form, which may have produced stigmata must also be obtained.

EXAMINATION

A full body examination should be performed. It is classically known that in the stress of a physical confrontation, symptoms of trauma, and memory of causation may be absent. This dictum is also true in the examination of a police officer in the case of alleged "police assault". The oft related habit of examining a constable's hands does a disservice to the profession and creates a two tier standard with a reduced level of competency for the police. To the police officer in such a situation should be extended the full facilities of a complete, competent and consensual examination.

The examination should be performed carefully. The order of the facets of the complete examination is completely at the discretion of the individual doctor, though developing a standard format and using proformata (see Chapter 4) can be helpful. It is important however, that any samples that should be obtained are taken at a time when they are not going to have been contaminated by previous procedures. This is particularly true in, but not exclusive to, sexual offences, and is covered in Chapters 8 & 9.

INJURIES

The recording of injuries accurately is absolutely vital.

The use of body charts (see Appendix 1c) is of great aid.

Any injury or lesion which can be measured, should be measured.

There are six objective parameters to any such traumatic lesion:

- Type of lesion
- Position
- Size
- Appearance
- Orientation
- Direction of causation

In addition to these there are the subjective symptoms of:

- Pain
- Tenderness
- Stiffness

These subjective findings should be recorded, but it must be noted and indicated in any report produced that these were elicited symptoms. It may be that experience will give the FME a good idea as to how genuine the symptom level was, but they, nevertheless, remain subjective.

TYPE OF LESION

The police surgeon is referred to the standard medical texts on these injuries for a full description. The description of these is particularly clear in *Clinical Forensic Medicine*, edited by Dr WDS McLay and published by Greenwich Medical Media this book is recommended reading.

A simple descriptive term should be applied wherever possible. A list of these terms follows, with an occasional note of caution or explanation.

Abrasion = Damage to the skin caused by tangential forces, may be dermal or only epidermal, often the latter can be extremely helpful in deciding on the direction of causation. Difficulty arises in the graduation from a deep abrasion to a wound. This is arbitrary but if the damage is deeper than the dermis, it may properly be called a wound. Caution should be exercised in calling an injury a wound, without consideration of the legal interpretation of "wounding"(v.i.).

Bruise = May be petechial, purpuric, larger (ecchymosis) or form a haematoma. The forensic clinician has a duty to use a term consistently and with a definitive meaning. Some may call a bruise ≤2mm in diameter a petechial haemorrhage, in which case they should always do so, others only if it is ≤1 mm. Explanation of such terms should be given in any report written (see page 39). Do remember that some lesions can be defined by palpation.

Scratch = May be considered an abrasion with length but no significant width, or a very superficial incision. The implication in describing a lesion as a scratch is that it was caused by a sharp point, or multiple points. Fingernail abrasions may have a measurable width, and if present it should be measured.

Incision = A sharp causation **never** to be confused with laceration.

Laceration = Caused by blunt force **never** to be confused with incision.[k]

Stab = A penetrating wound deeper than it is long.

Gunshot = Rifled, non-rifled, high velocity and low velocity weapons.

Burn = Friction, caustic, thermal.

---

k. However some wounds may have characteristics of both incisional cause and laceration and the varying components should be carefully recorded.

POSITION

The position of each injury should be noted. Not only should the area of the body be specified, such as describing it as being over the antero-lateral aspect of the left upper arm, but the distance the injury lies from a fixed point should be included. Fixed points on the body are recognisable bony protuberances, or from the floor with the body in a set position, e.g. standing.

It is often much easier to mark the approximate position on a body chart.

SIZE

The dimensions of an injury should be measured. This can occasionally cause problems as a single injury sometimes presents with multiple parts. Such lesions can be described as a collective, as long as interpretative elements are not lost by such a shorthand.

Measurements should use a single system. Ideally this should be metric.[1] The combination of inches and centimetres, for example, is not only confusing but appears casual and amateur. It would also be less likely to cause error if a single quantum is used. An example would be using 3 cm and 0.8 cm rather than 3 cm and 8 mm. Centimetres lend themselves readily to this. However the FME should use the quantum with which they are happy and familiar.

APPEARANCE

Any injury will have descriptive characteristics. Colour, shape and pattern should all be commented upon. A regular shaped, homogenously coloured bruise may offer more evidential value than irregular lesions.

The colour of a bruise may be used to ascertain its time since causation. Extreme caution must be employed. The work by Langlois & Gresham[70] would suggest that if yellow is visible in the bruise, it is more than 18 hours old. No other interpretation was deemed possible.

ORIENTATION

A slightly different facet from appearance, is orientation, of apparent axes of an injury, or aspect of curved lesions.

DIRECTION OF CAUSATION

This has been alluded to above under "Abrasion". On occasions certain aspects of an injury, such as varying depth, configuration of edges, or skin piling may

---

1. Many people, including some judges are still more familiar with imperial measures, and it is helpful to include these as well as metric or have a conversion table to hand.

suggest the direction in which the trauma applied itself to the tissue. On occasions this will be more readily seen with magnification, and every forensic clinician should have some means on hand to inspect an injury under magnification.

GENERAL NOTES

The use of definitive measurements is the norm. Description of lesion by reference to fruits, nuts or other flora is inaccurate and misleading, and should not therefore be used.

Though a good artist may wish to draw all the lesions on body charts, it is often just as easy to mark the approximate position on the chart, listing the dimensions and characteristics, alongside. If the lesions are many, numbering each one, not only allows for the text to be placed clear of the diagram, but is also a useful reference when constructing a statement.

Even if the physician lacks artistic talent, an injury displaying noticeable characteristics, such as an unusual or specific pattern should be drawn or photographed.

I reproduce here the paragraph from page 17 about photography but the clinician is referred to that chapter of the guidelines with regard to photography and consent.

Photographs can be useful as an adjunct to the handwritten records and/or sketches and are extremely useful as a teaching accessory later. Whenever possible a photograph of a lesion, as opposed to a scene, should contain a scale. **If photography is considered necessary for evidential purposes then the FME should contact the Senior Investigating Officer with regard to use of the professionally trained police photographer**. The use of photography as part of the clinical record should be a matter between the doctor and the patient alone. Only the latter has the right to consent (and/or parent if appropriate) and only the former is fit to judge whether it would be a useful way of recording part of the clinical record or useful for forensic education. Arguments have been offered to suggest that police surgeons should not take their own photographs, as these are essentially amateur by nature and may show discrepencies with any "official" photgraph. The argument progresses by suggesting that such photographs could be used adversely in any subsequent court case. Such an argument is fallacious so long as it is made clear that the photographs were only an adjunct to the written clinical records. The photograph should no more cause problems than should sketches made by the police surgeon.

A WOUND

In English law the term wound has a specific meaning. Though wounding is itself mentioned under section **18** & **20** of the Offences Against The Person Act 1861, the case law defining a wound predates this Act. In R _v_ M'Loughlin (1838) a wound was classified as having to have **broken the whole skin**. In the later case of R v Waltham (1849) **damage to the integrity of a mucous membrane** which was continuous with the skin could also constitute a wound.

It is therefore important for the FME to use the term wound with caution.

INVESTIGATIONS

As well as remembering that children of suspected physical abuse may need X-rays, it can be important to consider radiology as an investigative tool in adult cases.

The author has had radiological confirmation of a suspicion of pneumothorax in two cases of alleged victims of assault who claimed to have received hard blows to the thorax.

A paper from Edinburgh[71] was presented at the recent 5th Cross Channel Conference on Forensic Medicine, held in Paris in April 1995 which highlights another important area to consider. This paper illustrated a fracture of the greater horn of the hyoid bone in two survivors of attempted manual strangulation. Both were female and both had local symptoms.

Bite marks need to be photographed. A trained forensic odontologist should also be consulted. The views should be 1:1, with two scales at right angles, and three views perpendicular and either side at 45° in the same plane.

8

EXAMINATION OF VICTIM OF ALLEGED SEXUAL ASSAULT

EXAMINATION IN THE CASE OF ALLEGED SEXUAL ASSAULT

INTRODUCTION

There is no doubt that examinations of adults in this arena, along with those involving children, can be the most demanding of circumstances.

The first part of this chapter will deal with the adult. The second with the child where this differs.

This is not to say that other areas of clinical forensic medicine can be approached with less skill and more superficial knowledge; they cannot. In these areas however, the FME will be faced with establishing an ambience which will allow the necessary comprehensive examination to take place.

- Whilst preserving the dignity of the examinee as well as the forensic specimens

- By coaxing the patient to be compliant whilst allowing them to regain a control which may have been severely damaged during any assault

- Whilst accepting the patient's communications with total belief and compassion yet maintaining a scientific objectivity so that any evidence can be presented without bias or prejudice

"Examination" is a euphemism for the whole doctor/patient interface, involving as it does in good forensic practice, skills, knowledge and attitudes which go a long way beyond the ability to record genital findings.

Ideally the "processing" of a complainant, should take place within an organised structure involving not only appropriately trained and experienced forensic clinicians but also:

1. Trained police officers
2. Trained counsellors

3. Sexually Transmitted Disease (STD) screening facilities and specialist adviser.

4. Obstetric and Gynaecology /Urology /Paediatric specialist back up services

5. Specialist suites.

It is important that where possible the patient has a choice of gender of those who are going to have intimate contact with them.

In this chapter the use of the term "victim" must be read as "alleged victim". There is no intent that any forensic clinician should have a prejudicial bias. It is the court that will decide guilt or innocence, whatever the initial percieved truth of the matter.

Appendix 8a shows a schematic outline of Greater Manchester Services in this field.

GENERAL ISSUES

Medical records are important. Chapter 1 should be read.

Some centres (eg St Mary's Sexual Assault Centre (SMSAC) in Manchester) have developed their own proformata. If there are confidential notes or common notes which are important for continuing care such as counselling or STD treatment, it may be a policy that those notes are not removed from the centre. Otherwise the advice about record responsibility is as discussed in Chapter 1.

Consent has been covered in Chapter 2. Examination of a victim may present forensic and therapeutic aspects and the doctor must ensure that the appropriate informed consent is obtained. The police surgeon must be clear in his/her own mind before explaining the features of each to the examinee.

Though this chapter describes the situation with regard to females, the procedure apart from the obvious exception of the genital examination applies equally to male complainants. For examination of the penis, the section in the following chapter should be read.

It is extremely important that the patient understands that any relevant detail of the exchange between him/herself and the doctor may be discussed in public court.

THE EXAMINATION

Introduction

The FME should introduce him/herself, explaining what must be done.

The complainant should be asked how they would like to be addressed. It should not be assumed that they wish to be called by their first name.

Sympathy to their plight is important (remembering, but in no way expressing, that this predicament is only alleged at this stage), it can be expressed whilst the details of the thoroughness of the examination and sample taking procedure are explained. Attention should be drawn to the way the evidence can help in court, but additionally the examinee informed that no promises can be given as regards the outcome of any court case.

The benefit of being able to reassure as to the lack of anatomical damage can be comforting.

Explaining to the patient that they are in control, and even though the examination may be long and tedious, it should never be more than uncomfortable at the most and that they can call a halt at any time, may help to dispel some of the feeling of vulnerability which can be left after an assault.

Continuing to converse with or talk to the patient throughout the examination can be reassuring.

Specific medical problems can also be addressed such as STD. It is worth reminding the patient that this information is not recognised generally as being of value as forensic evidence, and that the disclosure is covered by law (see Chapter 3). If AIDS is mentioned as a specific concern, then it must be addressed in superficial general terms and specialist counselling arranged with pre and post HIV testing counselling sessions provided, otherwise it is best left for any counsellors to deal with it, if necessary, at a later date.

HISTORY OF EVENT

This should be obtained from the sources available. This usually means the reporting police officer and then the complainant. Detailed notes should be made and checked with the patient with particular reference to any discrepancies that exist between any versions received (see page 10 "WHAT").

A complainant may not mention all that has happened, and careful probing may be needed to elicit the full history of events (for example a female may be reluctant to admit buggery). Leading questions, as always, should be used as a last resort.

The history should also include recent sexual intercourse before and after the event.

GENERAL MEDICAL HISTORY

Current medical problems, and past medical, surgical, injury (not considered by some to be a medical problem) and obstetric & gynaecological history should be obtained.

Gynaecological history is important as is history of recent intercourse.

GENERAL EXAMINATION

The examination should be done using an appropriate sampling kit.

These are available commercially and contain all the relevant disposables for completing a forensic examination. These kits have been produced under the guidance of the Home Office Forensic Science experts as have the guidelines for the obtaining of specimens. Every police surgeon should be familiar with these forensic science guidelines.

Clothing – if the victim is wearing the original clothing this should be inspected for debris, damage, general condition, and orientation.[m] Semen should be specifically looked for by swabbing any sample that fluoresces under UV light. It should be remembered, however, that all that fluoresces is not semen by any means.

The clothes should be packaged according to forensic science instructions, each item wrapped separately, dry clothing in polybags and shoes in stout paper bags. Any damp item that is packaged must be transferred to the laboratory *without any delay* to avoid potentially rapid degradation of any organic evidence.

Damp knickers could be frozen.

Notes should be made of any areas of specific interest, and this information passed to the scientists.

The patient should have been undressed on a clean sheet of paper and any fallen debris thus collected. Rather than have the patient standing totally naked a suitable dressing gown could be provided, though the system should ensure that there is **no** chance of the dressing gown contaminating the evidence with fibres or debris unconnected with the case.

Record of any jewellery that was worn should be made.

Any samples or specimens collected by the police surgeon should be identified with a unique number for that case.

Standard procedure is for the clinician to use his/her initials with a number sequence.

It is important that if another examination is done, at another time, which is connected with the same case, the numbers are continued and not restarted at **"1"**, as this may, obviously, lead to confusion.

The samples and specimens should be handed to a police officer at the appropriate time, when all labelling has been fully completed and a note made of what samples were given to whom on what date and at what time. It is probably a safer practice to verbally indicate, as well as writing on the sample, any specific storage instructions to be followed. An example would be indicating which blood specimen (v.i.) should be frozen.

---

m. Was the clothing inside out or on in the wrong order?

Clinical features should all be recorded. Height, weight, general appearance and demeanour, as well as any fetor or other stigmata may all be important.

A thorough inspection of the body is necessary. The general body inspection can be done in sections to preserve the dignity of the patient as much as possible.

Any injury or significant lesion should be notated. See page 92 on examination in cases of assault.

Photography can be useful as an adjunct to the handwritten records and/or sketches and are extremely useful as a teaching accessory later. Whenever possible a photograph of a lesion, as opposed to a scene, should contain a scale. **If photography is considered necessary for evidential purposes then the FME should contact the Senior Investigating Officer with regard to use of the professionally trained police photographer**. It helps if female Scenes of Crime Officers (SOCOs) trained in evidential photography are available.

As well as the general injuries mentioned in the previous chapter there are further specific findings which may be of evidential value:-

Bite-marks, as well as photography and the referral to a forensic odontologist, should be swabbed. The swab should be moistened with water from a sterile ampoule, and twisted around on the bite area. If photography is performed without the presence of the odontologist the views should be ideally 1:1, with two scales at right angles, and three views perpendicular and either side at 45° in the same plane.

The eyes should be inspected for redness or petechiae.

The scalp may show petechiae, purpura or pin-point haemorrhage at the hair roots when the hair has been pulled. Hair loss may also be noted. The scalp should be palpated for soft tissue swelling.

The mouth should be inspected as should the auditory meatus and behind the pinnae.

It is possible that fellatio occurred causing petechiae on the palate.[72]

As well as soft tissue damage, the nails should be inspected for breaks or possible fibres or skin from the "assailant".

GENITAL EXAMINATION

The vulva should be inspected, under illuminated magnification, for redness, grazes, splits in the fourchette and bruising.

External swabs should be taken, including the peri-anal area.

Low vaginal swabs should be taken after gentle separation of the labia. Care must be taken not to introduce any external contaminant into the vagina.

A small (? "virgin sized") speculum should be carefully introduced. This should not be lubricated, except with water[n] but at a suitably warmed temperature.

Inspection of the internal walls of the vagina should then be done.

High vaginal swabs should then be taken, without touching the speculum or lower vaginal walls. At least two high vaginal swabs should be obtained. If there is obvious fluid present more swabs or a pipette could be used. In late presenting cases (more than 36 hours) an endo-cervical swab should also be taken. It may be necessary to use a larger speculum to visualise the cervix.

Recent work[73] has resulted in a single sperm being isolated from an endo-cervical swab after 14 days. With modern DNA amplification techniques, it is possible that suitable material may be obtainable after such a period when subjected to Polymerase Chain Reaction amplification.

Once the forensic swabs have been obtained, a more careful inspection of the whole vagina can be carried out. Occasionally a foreign body may be driven high into the posterior fornix, and any such material should be retrieved and sent for examination.

Finally a bimanual examination can be carried out, checking for any symptoms such as tenderness, or objective findings such as a gravid uterus.

STD specimens can then be taken with the patient's continued consent.

STD protocols should be developed and followed with the advice of a specialist in venereology.

The anus should be inspected. Swelling, bruising or fissures should be recorded. The anal opening should be described and any gaping or spasm noted. In appropriate cases an external anal swab having been taken (v.s.), the perianal area should be thoroughly cleansed with soap and water, then dried before any penetrative examination is performed. A small proctoscope can be inserted and the internal swabs obtained.

If the anus has been injured, the tenderness may be such that it is not possible to carry out such an examination at all, or only by using a lubricant. If a lubricant is used, this information should be passed on with the specimens, and a sample of the lubricant, to the forensic laboratory.

After due consideration, a digital examination can be done to test the tone of the anal sphincter.

A caring and sensitive approach will often allow a thorough anal examination.

If the examination is not thorough and no semen obtained from a high anal swab, it may not be possible to corroborate a charge of buggery. Equally if the

---

n. Consideration should be given as to whether tap water or sterile water is used. It appears that different specialist scientists have different opinions (no citations). It is the opinion of the panel preparing this document that sterile water should be used, until any published research proves it to be unnecessary.

clinician cannot guarantee the integrity of the high anal swab any charge of buggery may fail.

OTHER SPECIMENS

Pubic hair

After completing the above, the pubic hairs should be combed and any debris and loose hairs or other fibres collected along with the comb. The collected material including the comb should be securely fastened in an exhibit bag. Any matted areas of pubic hair should be cut off and sealed in a separate exhibit bag.

A small number of pubic hairs should be plucked (≤12) if needed.

Head hair

Head hair must be combed for debris and prepared as above.

Plucked head hairs should be obtained (about 25) and collected together in another exhibit bag. The sample should be obtained from various parts of the scalp.

Saliva and mouth

Saliva can be collected by asking the examinee to rinse out his/her mouth with a small amount of water and collecting the rinse in the bottle provided.

If there is any question of fellatio, then careful swabbing of the teeth may retrieve sperm, particular attention should be given to the interdental spaces and the gum margins.

Fingernails

Careful inspection of the fingernails may reveal fibres or other debris. The loose material and finger nail clippings should be gathered. Use one bag per hand, clipping/cutting the nails with the hand inside the bag. If the clipping is done outside the bag and the trajectory of the clipped fragment ends up on the floor, it is either lost or at risk of contamination.

Blood

Two samples of venous blood should be obtained for identification purposes. This should be placed in EDTA sample containers. Systems using the collecting bottle as the sample tube should be used. The common systems in use are Monovette and Vacutainer. Use the system that is provided in the "kit".

One sample should be frozen and labelled clearly as to the storage requirements, the other chilled.

Blood alcohol and drug assays should be considered if there is a reason to suspect either may be relevant to the case.

It is important to remember that the duty of the forensic clinician is to gather evidence impartially. The results, whether positive or negative, high or low may assist the case for the prosecution or defence. If the appropriate samples are not taken at the time, they are lost forever.

An alcohol estimation could be made using a breath analysis machine if one is available.

Skin

If a sample of "stain" (whether seen by fluorescence or not) on the skin is obtained, this should be done with a dry swab if moist, or a swab, itself moistened, using the sterile water ampoule in the kit, if dry. The same technique can be used for bite marks, or even if there is just a history of oral breast contact even in the absence of visible source material.

In such circumstances a control swab of an area of skin remote from the contamination should be obtained using the same supplies.

Specimen management

This involves labelling, documentation and disposal.

The specimens should be carefully checked. If the examination has to be performed without help, then the swab labelling should, ideally, be done beforehand.

The exhibit bags should be marked using a waterproof pen.

The documentation provided in any of the "kits" should be completed. This should provide a copy for the physician which will also act as the doctor's copy of the case identification legend.

Once the documentation is complete the specimens can be handed on to the person responsible for the next link in the chain to the laboratory. The time this exchange took place and the identity of the person taking the samples should then be added to the clinician's contemporaneous notes. It is also worth while drawing the receiver's attention to any specific instructions such as which specimens need to be frozen.

Control swabs should be provided including an unopened swab[o] The latter exhibit may not be used, but if not provided at the time, it will never be available.

---

o. In one case, involving the author, the unopened control swab in a case of arson (the swabs were of the hands in consideration of accelerants), was found to be contaminated with petroleum hydrocarbons! Presumably the swabs had been stored in the boot of a vehicle, or near a source of petroleum.

THERAPEUTIC AFTERCARE

The patient should have the opportunity to ask questions pertaining to the procedure undergone.

With the consent of the patient treatment, including Post Coital Contraception (PCC), if indicated, should be given or arranged, with appropriate follow up organised.

The officers in the case should be advised with regard to the patient's fitness to be interviewed, and the advice and considerations discussed in Chapter 6 on this subject should be read. In GMP, for example, the policy is not to interview in the middle of the night when the interviewee may be in shock, tired or intoxicated for example.

COMMUNICATIONS

A summary of the significant findings should be given to the investigating officer, with advice about their significance.

It is not improper for the clinician examining a complainant, to discuss, by telephone, any peculiar findings with the police surgeon examining the suspect.

Discussions have, apocryphally, attracted a condemnation of this practice as collusion. Such is not the case. There is no difference between giving the forensic scientist as much information as possible to enable him/her to carry out a professional analysis and extending the same courtesy to ones clinical colleagues. In all cases the clinician's role is to gather evidence which will help any court make a balanced decision.

CHILD ABUSE

Repeated here is a paragraph from the introduction:-

Continued professional development, keeping abreast of world literature and attending lectures and seminars is as important for the experienced physician as it is for the novice.

The novice should not be involved in examining children without the guide of an experienced clinician.

Children may present to the forensic clinician via a number pathways:

- Directly through the police
- From Social Services
- From Paediatric services
- From General Practitioners

Some Police Forces (GMP is one) agree that the benefit to the judicial process in having an experienced clinician involved at the beginning is such that those recognised to be competent in this field will be remunerated whatever the referral pathway. An extremely important advantage of this system is the ability for the number of examinations to which the child may be subjected to be reduced.

The specific areas relating to GMP are shown at Appendix 8b.

Child Physical Abuse often presents via hospital and will be investigated by hospital based services without an FME being involved. Where the police surgeon is called in, the detail of injuries should be recorded as laid out on page 92. Particular attention should be made to

- Injuries of different ages
- Areas of special significance, eg inside the lip, and behind the ear
- Radiological expertise should be sought if at all indicated.

Where a child is seen in hospital, the forensic clinician should also make entries in the hospital notes as well as their own contemporaneous record. Naturally the factual information recorded should be identical, even if presented in a different format. Discrepancies in the different records of the findings from a single practitioner may result in the evidence failing in court. If a joint examination is made the practitioners should agree on the findings. If there is a lack of concurrence about a lesion such a finding should be notated.

Joint examinations can occur in both physical and sexual abuse cases for a number of reasons. A Paediatrician may not lack the forensic skills but wishes to concentrate on the therapeutic aspects leaving the forensic implications to a skilled doctor remote from the care aspect and the family.

Joint opinion can also add weight to the presentation in court.

CHILD SEXUAL ABUSE

Unlike physical abuse, alleged Child Sexual Abuse (CSA) does not necessarily need an urgent examination. Often the abuse has occurred over an extended period of time and there is no forensic evidence to be lost.

However, in the case of "stranger" molestation, the rapidity of the examination may prove crucial to the preservation of trace evidence.

Even though there is often no scientific urgency, the child and his family are in a situation of great stress which may be alleviated to some extent by the calm professional approach of the doctor.

There may also be some constraints under PACE if a suspect is in police custody. It is often of importance for the investigating officers to have information obtained in the medical examination before they interview the suspect.

For these reasons the examination should be conducted as speedily as is reasonable.

Consent

Consent is covered in Chapter 2, however there are some special considerations to be addressed with regard to minors.

Though it is not necessary in law for consent to be obtained from a young child, as it is unlikely that the child would understand all the ramifications of such an examination, no child should be forcibly examined.

The only exception would be a crying toddler who might be held firmly on his-mothers knee whilst a general inspection was done.

As a general rule a child should not be examined without parental consent as well.

If medical examination is considered necessary and the parent(s) refuses consent, legal advice should be sought. Application can be made to the Court for:-

i Emergency Protection Order with directions in a child protection situation
ii Specific Issue Order (This is covered on page 18.)

Who can give consent?

i if the child is the subject of Police Protection, the police do not have parental responsibility, and consent should be sought from the parent(s).
ii if the child is subject to a Child Assessment Order, the Local Authority does not have parental responsibility. The Court will give directions regarding examination etc.
iii if the child is subject to an Emergency Protection Order (sec **44** Children Act 1989), the applicant (usually Local Authority) has parental responsibility. The Court has power to direct medical or psychiatric examination or assessments of the child, or direct that there be no such examination etc.

History

The FME should obtain details of the alleged offence from the police officer and/or social worker and make appropriate notes.

The child must not be interviewed in depth as there are strict rules about the way that such interviews are conducted.[74]

If it came to the notice of the Court that the child had been questioned in detail by the doctor, it is possible that the child's evidence would be regarded as contaminated and inadmissible.

If questions have to be asked at all about the allegations they should be non-leading questions.

Children over the age of 12 years have been shown to be no more suggestible than adults and have a similar ability at recall.

Sometimes children are seen with a genital injury which has stimulated suspicion amongst medical personnel, such as a child being brought to casualty. A proper history from the carers and the child might well resolve the matter quickly if the injury is consistent with the mechanism blamed.

Introduction

After introductions to the child and accompanying persons the appropriate consent should be obtained.

Explain what is to happen and invite the co-operation of the child. Older children should have some choice about who is present in the examination room. Reassurance should be given that the child has control and can stop, if becoming distressed.

A general history should be obtained with particular note of any condition which may confuse the issue of signs of abuse.

Examination

The examination must be tailored to each individual case.

The child who has been indecently touched, but no more, by a family member should in no circumstances be subjected to a detailed medical examination which may be perceived, by the child, to be more intrusive than the alleged offence. Equally a perfunctory examination which fails to reveal evidence which is present is also detrimental to the welfare of the child.

The police surgeon must carefully assess the facts, decide on what procedures need to be undertaken, make good records and be prepared to justify those decisions under cross-examination in court.

In the case of a serious sexual assault the procedure outlined above in relation to the adult should be followed.

The examination should proceed at a pace suitable for the comfort of the child. Talking to the patient helps.

Starting the examination by weighing and measuring, and performing general medical tests such as otoscopy all help to put the child at ease with what, for many, are familiar procedures.

The findings should be recorded on percentile and Tanner charts. Failure to thrive and dips in the normal growth projection can be associated with abuse.

A full examination and record of any lesion can follow.

GENITAL EXAMINATION IN GIRLS

A small child is often most easily examined on her mother's knee, particularly if only a visual inspection is needed. The mother can hold the child's legs apart. Alternatively a similar inspection can be done with the child lying prone over the mother's knee with the clinician examining from behind.

With older children, the usual technique is for the child to be examined lying supine on the medical couch with her knees flexed and hips externally rotated. Whilst in this position the labia may be gently separated (labial separation) by the examiner's fingers or traction exerted in a forward and downward direction with the examiner holding the labia gently between thumb and forefinger (labial traction).

The genital area can also be examined thoroughly with the child in the knee-chest position.[p] In this position the important posterior edge of the hymen can often be seen more clearly than when the child is lying supine on the couch.

Ideally the child should be examined in both positions. The child should however be given control over the choice. Many children appear to prefer the knee chest position.

Ideally a colposcope should be used, but in the absence of this a magnifying glass or optical loups are an alternative. The colposcope should include optical measurement and recording.

In many cases when the genitalia are examined in different positions, the edge of the hymen will have been clearly visualised without the need for any kind of intrusive examination, but in some cases it is helpful to use a glass probe (Glaister's globe).

Glaister's globes are glass rods with a diameter of 0.6 mm with one end of the rod being expanded into a globe from 1–2.5 cm in diameter. They can be inserted gently behind the hymen to display its edges over the glass. In this way apparent folds and indentations often smooth out and small nicks and tears can be more easily identified. Glass rods used in this way, with explanation and demonstration to the child, are much less traumatic than using a moistened cotton wool swab which often causes pain in a delicate area.

If swabs have been taken for forensic purposes, or to carry out tests for STD, then it is helpful to show the child an unused swab. In some cases it helps to allow the child to use the swab herself and keep control. Again the child should be allowed to halt the proceedings if distressed.

In most cases where indecent acts are alleged it is not necessary, after the above procedures, to insert any object into the vagina. However, where there is an allegation of full sexual intercourse or findings such as a completely torn hymen,

---

p. Crouched on the examination couch with the small of the back arched downwards, knees flexed under the chest and bottom in the air.

then in some cases it is appropriate to carry out a gentle digital examination of the vagina to establish whether:

- The hymenal ring is completely torn
- Whether the vagina can admit an object the size of an erect penis and
- Whether its walls are rugose or smooth and the canal enlarged

In older girls it may be appropriate to carry out a full gynaecological examination, including the insertion of a speculum, to inspect the cervix. Bimanual palpation may indicate pregnancy and a pregnancy test may be advisable.

GENITAL EXAMINATION IN BOYS

There is rarely any genital injury in boys who have been indecently assaulted. The penis and testicles should be thoroughly inspected for signs of bruising, tears of the frenulum, or "love-bites" and signs of sucking. The root of the penis may show bruising or other lesions. It is important to consider that the penis may have been sucked and to swab for saliva, in the knowledge that saliva, on the unwashed penis, may survive for up to one week.

The testicles should be examined for signs of bruising or biting.

The anal area

The anus should be inspected in every case. This may be done in the left lateral or knee-chest position.

The buttocks should be gently separated, without applying traction, and the anal orifice observed for about 30 seconds to see if there is any dilatation. Slight twitchiness or dilatation of the external sphincter is probably of no significance. Anal dilatation in the presence of a stool in the rectum is regarded by most experienced examiners as being unlikely to be a sign of abuse. If observed, however, it should be recorded.

The anal folds should be regular and symmetrical around the anal opening but there is often a redundant fold, particularly in boys, anteriorly which can be confused with a skin tag or healed fissure. A midline raphe extending backwards from the scrotum is normal and should not be confused with signs of injury.

Prominent veins have sometimes been claimed to be significant pointers to abuse. However, they often come up during the examination as the child tenses and relaxes his muscles, and no great significance can be attached to them, though they must, of course, be noted.

If no abnormality is seen on careful inspection of the anus then it is appropriate to do no more. However if there is an allegation of anal abuse then a finger gently can be placed against the anal orifice to test its tone. A very good estimate of anal tone can be obtained in this way without doing a full digital examination. In some cases a digital examination should be done, the subject asked to squeeze the examining finger to test the anal tone. It is important to remember, however, that this procedure relies on a subjective assessment of the examiner based on experience and can be unreliable.

POINTS TO REMEMBER

1. The majority of children where sexual abuse is alleged will present no objective signs

   1.1 As there was no intention to hurt the child physically

   1.2 And the abuse may have occurred some time earlier

2. It is difficult to differentiate the normal from the abnormal. Increasing research particularly in the USA has demonstrated a much greater variations in the normal than was previously believed. Such that:-

   2.1 A view put forward in the 1980s that 0.4 cm was the upper limit of the hymenal orifice in a non-abused child has been shown, by careful study of apparently non-abused children to be incorrect; a rough working guide to this diameter would be 1 mm per year of age

3. There are excessive claims for the value of medical evidence and forensic clinicians must guard against trying to fit the evidence to the case. This type of behaviour has all too often led to medical evidence being discredited in Court. Total objectivity from the beginning of the case will save much investigative time, and more importantly save the child being let down at a later date in Court

4. The questions that must be answered are

   4.1 If the findings occurred in a child where no allegation of abuse existed would suspicion be raised anyway?

   4.2 Do the findings commonly occur in abused children?

   4.3 What is the mechanism resulting in the "abnormal" finding?

SEXUALLY TRANSMITTED DISEASE

In most cases, in children, tests for sexually transmitted disease are not done. If there are genital symptoms, or the child or parents are worried, then tests can be done after any forensic specimens have been obtained. The protocol of the local laboratory that will analyse the specimens should be followed.

A request for testing for HIV should stimulate advice and referral to specialist counselling services.

REASSURANCE

Reassurance in CSA is one of the more important roles that the FME can play.
Reassurance that no physical defects will result from whatever happened.
Reassurance that whatever did happen was not the fault of the child.

9

EXAMINATION OF SUSPECT IN SEXUAL ASSAULT

EXAMINATION OF SUSPECT IN SEXUAL ASSAULT

This chapter is short.

The brevity with which this particular aspect of FME work has been treated is inversely proportional to its importance.

The two previous Chapters (7 & 8) need to be read.

The standard of detail with which a specific suspect needs to be examined is no less than in the examination of an alleged victim.

The forensic clinician owes a duty to accused, victim and the courts to perform a thoroughly professional appraisal.

If the alleged offence is remote from the examination of the suspect, such that weeks have passed, it may not be worthwhile looking for forensic material other than blood for identification.

It should be remembered that bruises may be visible for 14 days.[70] They may be visualised with specialist UV photography (mainly of benefit in bite-marks) for up to 4 months.[75]

If a particular scar, skin lesion or other distinguishing mark has been mentioned by the complainant, it may be appropriate to perform an inspection whatever the delay.

Repeated here is the opinion emphasised in the previous chapter.

It is not improper for the clinician examining the suspect, to discuss, by telephone, any peculiar findings with the police surgeon examining a complainant.

Discussions have, apocryphally, attracted a condemnation of this practice as collusion. Such is not the case. There is no difference between giving the forensic scientist as much information as possible to enable him/her to carry out a professional analysis and extending the same courtesy to ones clinical colleagues. In all cases the clinician's role is to gather evidence which will help any court make a balanced decision.

PROCEDURE

Discuss with the Senior Investigating Officer (SIO) the purposes of the examination. No forensic clinician should be satisfied with a request to simply "get blood and hair samples please". Full discussion should take place about the complexities of the case and then the police surgeon should inform the SIO about the extent and restrictions of any examination. The FME should also ensure that the appropriate requirements for the obtaining of intimate samples (v.i.) have been fulfilled.

The suspect should have the right to be seen without the presence of a police officer. Though as has been mentioned previously in the guidelines, the custody officer may object to this if there is a safety consideration.

If the suspect wishes the solicitor to be present, then this should pose no problem. However undue delay should not be contemplated at the risk of losing forensic evidence. Fibre evidence, for example, may degrade within a few hours.

Written consent should be obtained. This should include in the dialogue a mention of why the examination is being performed. An example would be "in the case of an alleged rape". The examination structure and sample procedure should be outlined. The disclosure pathways should be mentioned (see Chapters 2 & 3).

If consent is refused, then the police surgeon can still make observations and record those findings.

INTIMATE SAMPLES

If intimate samples are required then consent under PACE requirements which includes the written consent of the examinee will already have been obtained.[76] This should not deter the clinician from obtaining his/her own consent. A simple explanation that such consent is a medical ethic rather than a legal requirement usually produces amicable compliance.

Intimate samples are defined under Police and Criminal Evidence Act 1984 **s65** as amended by the Criminal Justice and Public Order Act 1994 **s58**

Intimate samples are:-

- Dental impression
- Sample of blood
- Sample of semen
- Any other tissue fluid
- Urine
- Pubic hair
- Swab from a body orifice other than the mouth.

With the exception of urine, none can be taken by anyone other than a registered dental or medical practitioner.

Having obtained consent, a history of the alleged incident should be requested. As many allegations relate to the question of consent or what actually occurred rather than the identification of who the perpetrator was this is not as fruitless as it may at first seem.

Sometimes, however, no event related history is forthcoming.

The examination should proceed.

A sexual offences kit should be used and, unless the clothes have already been obtained by the police, the examinee undressed on a paper sheet as with a victim. The clothes should be carefully packaged and the same courtesy of dignity extended to the patient as is given to the victim.

Clinical findings and the sample harvest should be performed meticulously and recorded accurately.

If injuries are discovered duing the examination, the examinee can be asked to account for them, even if no history was obtained, and even if legal advice, or the patient himself results in no response. The police surgeon should record "no response" without expression or comment and carry on with the procedure. Though "comments " should not be made, it is good clinical practice to maintain a discourse with the examinee throughout the contact, even if only in so far as explaining exactly what is entailed in the examination process. However the doctor should not embark on an interrogation that should properly be conducted by the investigating officer.

The genital examination should be as gentle as possible but thorough. The area, as with the rest of the body should be viewed under UV light for fluoresence, and any stain swabbed. Even in the absence of fluorescence a swab should be taken of the coronal sulcus.

The anal and peri-anal area should be inspected and examined in more detail depending on the allegations and findings. Though it must be remembered that consent may be witheld for any individual part of the examination process, and such a decision must be respected.

At the end of the examination it could be advantageous to ask the suspect and particularly the solicitor, if present, if they have any comment or criticism to voice. Record any answer.

The samples should be labelled in the same manner as described in Chapter 8 and also disposed of similarly.

10

THE SCENE
OF DEATH

THE DOCTOR AT
THE SCENE OF DEATH

INTRODUCTION

Police surgeons get called to many scenes of death.

The majority will not become the scene of a major crime investigation.

It is imperative that the clinician brings his/her skills and knowledge to the scene, alert from the beginning. It is likely that the police surgeon is the only one present with the medical and scientific training to perceive some anomalies which may give rise to suspicion.

FMEs are usually called to a death, because it is "suspicious", sudden or the General Practitioner of the deceased is unknown or not contactable. Suspicious deaths, in this context, are likely to include homicide, suicide or accidents, as well as some cases of natural death.

This chapter is not intended to be a panorama of death and its forensic aspects but to draw attention to the main areas of consideration.

These are:-

1. Approach to the scene
2. Communication
3. FMEs actions at the scene
4. Safety

All police surgeons should be familiar with the Scenes of Crime Directive produced by their Police or by the Home Office Forensic Science Laboratories (or the Metropolitan Service).

APPROACH TO THE SCENE

Contamination of the scene should be avoided.

The only exception to a slow measured and controlled approach to a body is the possibility that the life may be preserved in which case the primary responsibilty is the patient. Such preservation should not be undertaken without first making sure the scene is without danger to the doctor or others (see "Safety" below).

Approaching the scene of death, the doctor should alight from his/her transport no closer than the nearest police vehicle, unless directed to a particular area by a uniformed police officer or other official. It may appear that some vehicle is closer to the scene, but that may be one that is connected with the death.

If the FME is only the second or third person to arrive, he should discuss with the reporting officer the circumstances of the case before inspecting the body, and determine life to be extinct with as little disturbance to the scene as possible. If it is early in the case, or there may need to be an investigation, the police surgeon should not hesitate to inform his police colleagues about protection of the scene and the prevention of intrusion by unwanted observers.

If an investigation team is already there, it is likely that one officer will be keeping the log. The doctor should report his/her arrival to that log-keeper. Discussion with the Senior Investigating Officer (SIO) or equivalent should occur to determine the path of entry to the body and the known circumstances. The FME should keep to this path, which should be marked, with tape or stepping plates, where necessary.

The metaphor that it is best to keep ones hands in ones pocket should be taken literally. If without pockets, thinking about this adage should be enough to keep ones hands away from anything other than the body.

Having determined that life is extinct, no further interference with the body should take place without clearance from the SIO, and until after the Scenes of Crime Officers (SOCO) have completed their evidence gathering from the undisturbed body and environs. If the case is one without suspicion and no investigation is taking place it is still good practice for the professionals there to be informed before the doctor moves the body. In these latter circumstances, if the doctor is intending to take photographs for his/her clinical records, they should also be started before moving the body.

It is good practice, even in the most obvious and benign cases, for the body to be inspected on all sides, just in case a suspicious lesion or object lurks beneath.

The doctor should exit by the agreed pathway.

In the case of suspicious deaths, the doctor should remain, whenever possible, to offer to the investigating team his/her expertise, until the Home Office Pathologist arrives, or the body is removed. It is educational, *if ever case load permits*, for the clinician to attend the autopsy if possible.

COMMUNICATION

Good communication skills are an important part of the forensic clinicians armament at any time but are particularly useful at the scene of death.

It does not help to be imperious no matter how busy. The agreed procedures should be followed. As well as informing the investigating team of your presence and confirming death, the police surgeon has a lot to offer from a clinical aspect. The SIO should make use of the FME's skills and knowledge.

If the death is not considered to be other than natural and the FME is unhappy about the circumstances, then it is important for the doctor to communicate this dis-ease.

The police surgeon should not need to inform the Coroner as this will be done via the police services.

But it must be remembered that any death which cannot be registered falls under the jurisdiction of the Coroner.

The doctor should keep adequate notes relating to the death, including the identity of the SIO or reporting officer, time of arrival and time of confirmation of death.

In the case of criminal investigation, accidents may happen, if the doctor deviates from the agreed approach, or disturbs the scene, it does not help to conveniently forget the mishap. Report it. Rather than be criticised, it is likely to be appreciated and may save many man hours of searching for a footprint or fingerprint which belonged to the local divisional police surgeon.

Some scenes, fires and road traffic accidents are two examples, may involve other emergency services with their own skills to offer and responsibilities to serve, it is good practice to discuss matters with their senior representatives at the scene, if only from a safety angle.

ACTIONS AT THE SCENE

First do not become a victim (see "SAFETY" page 128).

Confirmation of death

This may be made by observation, assessing the absence of cardiopulmonary activity, loss of corneal reflex, "training" of retinal vessels etc.

The minimum to satisfy that life is extinct should be done initially, but the physician must be so satisfied.

If appropiate the body may be examined. The FME should be sensitive to signs which are anamolous to the apparent situation.

Unless resuscitation is an option any neck ligature, noose or tie should not be untied. If the body is suspended it should be cut down, once the scene has been assessed, with the "rope" being severed away from the knot.

Presentation and patterns

These aspects of injury play an important part in this. Some examples follow.

In the case of suicidal hanging,
- Was it possible for the deceased to have set up the suspension apparatus?
- Does the impression mark of the "noose" or "tie" lead to an appropriate suspension point?

In the case of any death,
- Does any livor or rigor mortis suggest the body was moved?

With bruising,
- Could it have been accidental?
- Were the "triangles of safety"q affected?
- Are petechiae, if present, in an appropriate distribution for the manner of death, or, if post-mortem, confined to areas of lividity sparing pressure areas of blanched skin?
- Is the lesion a bite-mark? if so specialist photography is needed. The views should be ideally 1:1, with two scales at right angles, and three views-pendicular and either side at 45° in the same plane.

In the case of tissue trauma,
- Were the lesions post-mortem?
- Could tissue loss be due to animal damage?

Time since death

Timing the moment of death has always been of great interest. The forensic clinician is urged to read *The Estimation of the Time Since Death in the Early Postmortem Period* edited by Professor Bernard Knight and published by Edward Arnold in 1995 (ISBN 0 340 57319 8). Even this tome will not give a definitive answer. In the Preface Bernard Knight writes " This book does not pretend to solve this ancient difficulty, but offers a series of monographs by different authors, which address various aspects of the problems".

If asked to give a time of death, the FME should always ask "why does it need to be known?" If it is not important do not interfere with the body more than necessary until the Forensic Pathologist has had his/her chance to inspect the unadulterated scene.

The police surgeon should be aware, however of the various methods by which estimates of the time of death can be made, and those factors which can influence the calculations.

Body temperature – Core temperature is needed. The reliability of rectal temperature was questioned as long ago as 1949.[77] In addition, if there is any question of sexual assault, the ano-genital area should not be contaminated except under careful controlled conditions and only then after carefully gathering any other forensic evidence.

---

q. Such as within the orbit, under the angle of the jaw, at sides of larynx.

The temperature at time of death, ambient temperature, climate changes since death, position and state of clothing of body, and whether the body was in wet or dry surroundings can all affect body cooling. The Henssge Normogram is probably the most sophisticated system for using temperature for time since death estimation and is well covered in the book mentioned above and referenced here.[78] The tables accompanying the normogram allow the observer to make allowance for most of the varying conditions mentioned above. If the police surgeon wishes to estimate time of death, he/she should familiarise themselvs with a suitable technique and then use that technique regularly.

Body fluid chemistry changes – Electrolyte concentrations in vitreous humour is the common one considered. Potassium is the main one estimated, but does require accurate technique and subsequent laboratory analysis and should not be done without reference to the pathologist who may wish to take a sample from the other eye later, though there is doubt as to whether this adds to the accuracy.[79] Potassium levels tend to rise after death in the vitreous humour, but an accurate sampling technique is crucial.

Lividity – Lividity is very variable, although helpful from some aspects (see reference to bruising on previous page) it should not be used for time estimations.

Rigor mortis – When possible all FMEs should familiarise themselves with the feeling of post-mortem rigidity. There are many variable factors. Complete rigidity generally can take from 6-20 hours to develop, but may persist much longer.[78]

Forensic entomology – Can help but does need expert analysis. The expert will focus on many arthropoda and not just insect identification and metamorphosis. If insect larvae are to be preserved, placing them in boiling water, or at a temperature of at least 60°C is the method to be used.[80]

Ancillary factors

Other factors are often more helpful with estimating the approximate time of death and may also help with the circumstances of the death.

- When was the deceased last seen alive?
- If at home is the calender marked off ?
- Mail, newspapers, milk deliveries and other dateable consumables may all aid the calculations.
- Are the curtains normally always opened at a certain time?
- Is there sign of a particular meal having been consumed?

It often falls to the police surgeon to speak to relatives. This can be an uncomfortable encounter with patients unknown to the doctor, especially when suicide or particularly auto-erotic accidental death is concerned as they will often have many questions. Answering some of these questions must be resisted when they

require a prediction of the official cause of death, an area which is the preroga-
tive of the Coroner (or Procurator Fiscal).

Mass disasters

These should evoke a predetermined formula from police forces. It is not
unusual for the divisional police surgeon to be one of the first on the scene. As
well as the obvious benefit of having the skills of a physician for the injured, the
FME can also aid in the identification of human remains. The preservation of
life and the reduction of post traumatic morbidity being the primary responsibilities, any other involvement should be done in an organised fashion under the
direction of the scene co-ordinator.

SAFETY

Some scenes are hazardous.

The police surgeon has a duty to protect officers or others present but more
important not to become a casualty him/herself.

Apart from the obvious environmental problems of building sites or precipitous
locations other hazards exist.

In death by electrocution the doctor should ensure that the power supply to the
body is not live.

Two bodies together should always alert the FME to the possibility of Carbon
Monoxide poisoning, but a single corpse may have died from similar cause.

It is sensible to carry protective clothing and suitable footwear for all terrains and
conditions.

QUICK REFERENCE

- Ensure body is dead
- Do not become a casualty
- Talk to the team
- Offer advice
- Do not contaminate the scene

11

MENTAL HEALTH

MENTAL HEALTH

The police surgeon will be called out to many problems relating to mental health.

The call-out will be usually as a consequence of:

- **s136** of the Mental Health Act 1983(MHA)
- Abnormal behaviour of a detainee
- Requirement of fitness for interview.

THE MENTAL HEALTH ACT

There are nine sections of the MHA which directly impinge on the FME; they are:

1 **Section 1** which defines

   1.1 "mental disorder"

   1.2 "severe mental impairment"

   1.3 "mental impairment" and

   1.4 "psychopathic disorder"

   1.5 and which, in subsection (3) protects promiscuity, immoral conduct, sexual deviancy or dependence on alcohol or drugs from the umbrella of this act, if existing alone.

2 **Section 2** which allows compulsory admission and detention to hospital

   2.1 For assessment

   2.2 On the recommendation of two doctors

   2.3 For up to 28 days

   2.4 Because of a mental disorder which

   2.5 Is in the interests of the health and safety of the patient or others.

3 **Section 3** which allows compulsory admission and detention to hospital

   3.1 For treatment

3.2   On the recommendation of two doctors?

3.3   For up to 6 months (s20)

3.4   Because of any of the definitions above (but must be with a view to treatment being likely to work in the case of "mental impairment" or "psychopathic disorder",

3.5   Is in the interests of the health and safety of the patient or others

3.6   And such treatment cannot be provided without admission

4   **Section 4** which allows compulsory admission to hospital

    4.1   In an emergency

    4.2   On the recommendation of one doctor

    4.3   For 72 hours

    4.4   For same reasons as 2.5

5   **Section 11** defines

    5.1   The applicant as nearest relative or approved social worker (ASW)

    5.2   and the documentary procedure.

6   **Section 12** defines the status of the doctors involved

    6.1   The doctors must complete the documentation not later than the date of admission

    6.2   They must have examined the patient together or within 5 days of each other

    6.3   One of the doctors must have been approved by the Secretary of State as having special experience in the diagnosis or treatment of mental disorder

    6.4   And the other doctor should know the patient unless the "approved" doctor fits that description?

    6.5   Sets prohibitions of who may be the "applicant"

7   **Section 135** allows a constable

    7.1   After an application by an ASW to a justice

    7.2   To enter, using force if necessary, any specified premises

    7.3   To remove a person believed

    7.4   To be suffering from a mental disorder

    7.5   Who suffers ill-treatment, neglect or lack of control or

    7.6   Lives alone and is unable to care for himself

    7.7   To a place of safety

    7.8   **or** Allows a constable

    7.9   After an application by a constable, or other authorised person, to a justice

    7.10   To enter, using force if necessary, any specified premises

7.11 To remove a person believed to be liable to MHA (or **s83** Mental Health (Scotland) Act 1960).

7.12 To a place of safety

7.13 For up to 72 hours.

8 **Section 136** allows a constable

8.1 To remove to a place of safety

8.2 For 72 hours

8.3 From a public place

8.4 A person who appears to be suffering from a "mental disorder"

8.5 And who needs immedicate care and control.

9 **Section 118** allows the Secretary of State to produce a Codes of Practice

In this chapter and Chapter 6 on Fitnees to be Interviewed, when referring to the codes of practice in general, the PACE codes will be referred to as Codes (PACE) and the Codes of Practice of the Mental Health Act 1983 will be referred to as Codes (MHA). All sections will be hereafter marked as "s" followed by the number.

The Codes (PACE) demand certain levels of response for a mentally disordered or handicapped person in custody.

Any person detained under **s136** MHA should be assessed as soon as possible and an ASW and medical practitioner should be called as soon as possible.

Once interviewed and examined and suitable arrangements have been made the patient can no longer be detained at the police station.

On occasions finding a suitable place for the patient to go whether it be a hospital bed or local authority address is difficult. Though not appropriate for either the patient or the custody staff, the patient can be kept up to 72 hours (v.s. 8.2 above).

If the person is to be released, that should not happen until he has been interviewed by both medical practitioner and ASW. If care is not required but the patient is to be interviewed in a criminal matter, an Appropriate Adult (AA) should be called. If the police officers involved have been so concerned as to bring in the patient under **s136** it would seem sensible to indicate that an AA must be called, unless the detainee had been acting.

The Codes (MHA), most recently published in August 1993, refer to other considerations.

Where the police station is to be the place of safety, the removal is to be treated as an "arrest" for the purposes of PACE and therefore Codes (PACE) in their entirety apply.

Section 10.2 of the Codes (MHA) state that:

" the local implementation policy should ensure that the doctor examining the patient should wherever possible be "approved"". The "approved" refers to s12 approval.

If learning disabilities are suspected then the advice is that it is desirable that the physician is a consultant psychiatrist in this field and the ASW has experience of such work.

One of the great difficulties with regard to **s136** is that there are no formal registration facilities, or record kept of how often it is used.

The PACE record would show that pathway as being the origin of the patient, and if referred on to hospital the clinical details will also show it. If the patient is released from custody there is no accesible register.

Many detainees are brought in to the custody situation for a "Breach of the Peace" and only when there is time to reflect does it appear that there may be a mental disorder.

In one survey[81] out of 872 consecutive patients only 41 (4.7%) were due to mental disorder (including s136). Of those only 13 (1.5%) needed hospital admission for assessment.

The 13 admitted represent only 31.7% of the total number seen.

Of the rest 16 remained in custody, 8 were released and 4 were referred to social services accomodation.

If this survey is represenatative it can be seen that nearly 70% of the "mental disorder" work would not result in acute specialist input.

This is not to say that the rest were without psychiatric morbidity. It seems unnecessary for Specialist Psychiatric Services to be involved at the police station in the first instance, but the recommendation for the primary physician to be "approved" is obviously valid.

Similar to Chapter 5 Fitness to be Detained, there is no intention for this chapter to be a textbook of Psychiatry.

There are important aspects to the care and treatment of mental disorder in the custody situation and the forensic clinician should keep up to date with continuing medical education in this field.

Diversion panels, to deal more appropriately with mentally disordered offenders, are becoming the norm since the Reed report was published.[82] It is important that forensic clinicians establish communications with these diversionary panels, if not already a member.

Those patients already on medication need to be carefully assessed. The General Practitioner and Consultant Psychiatrist who know the patient should be contacted where practicable.

Care must be taken with medication. Local case reports (unpublished) of severe extrapyramidal signs have occurred with moderate doses of phenothiazines. If phenothiazines are used, caution must be exercised over the dose. Anti-muscarinic drugs are not recommended prophylactically but if the patient is on them they should be continued.

It must be remembered that depression and alcoholism each offer significantly increased risk of suicide.

FORMAL REFERRAL TO HOSPITAL

In the case of deciding a detainee has a mental illness for which compulsory admission to hospital is required the FME should be familiar with the local arrangements.

Ideally the FME will be **s12** approved, the ASW and Consultant Psychiatrist will see the patient and admission under **s2** (or **s3**) can be arranged. It is not considered appropriate for an admission to be arranged under **s4** unless clinical urgency really does exist. If the patient is a detainee in custody it is difficult to see how the clinically urgent admission could be appropriate.

The gathering of the necessaary professionals can take some time. Though it is an advantage to meet together, it is not mandatory. There is often no need for the police surgeon to wait at the police station until the procedure is completed. Forms can be filled in and left or the police surgeon can arrange to return when the others are available.

The forensic clinician should keep accurate clinical records as well as completing the appropriate documents as demanded by the MHA.

The case of violent or dangerous patients poses difficult problems. Secure beds are not in great supply and admission except by court order normally relies on arrangements between General Psychiatric services and Forensic Psychiatric services to which police surgeons have no direct access. These cases can be very time consuming, but the custody officers needs the positive support of the police surgeon whilst arrangements are made. If the FME leaves the patient in custody whilst awaiting return messages, it is good practice to keep the custody officer informed of the progress, or lack of it, periodically.

12

ROAD TRAFFIC OFFENCES

ROAD TRAFFIC OFFENCES

INTRODUCTION

The forensic clinician enters a complex world in his/her dealings with the Road Traffic Acts (RTA) where a knowledge of driver statute and case law may be more important than in any other field.

At first it seems simple, that the FME is called out, turns up, takes blood samples and fills in some forms, and for the vast majority of cases that is the end of the matter.

It is for the few cases which are not simple that a wider knowledge is required.

RTA case law is full of examples where procedure rather than simple fact has been the lynch pin of a defended case.

By the "RTA", in this text, reference is being made to the Road Traffic Act 1988, the last in a series of Acts. The latter act is the source of virtually all the discussion in this chapter. Any other statute will be cited and described with its full title, but otherwise RTA will mean the '88 Act.

TECHNICAL MATTERS

The current RTA kits involve the doctor transferring blood from a single syringe to two containers with a "rubberised" membrane through which the blood can be injected. It is hard to conceive of any other procedure in medical practice today which is designed to be as hazardous to the user from the point of view of needle-stick injury or aerosol blood spray as this.

In 1994, a sub-committee of the Association of Police Surgeons met with representatives of the Home Office Forensic Science Services to address this problem amongst others. There appeared to be no problem in attitude from the scientists with regard to the re-organisation necessary for analysis using a different and safer venesection process. However the legal advice sought suggested that any other system available whereby two samples were obtained could not be deemed to have satisfied the Road Traffic Offenders Act 1988 **s15** (5)ʳ until it had been through the courts. It was not satisfactory therefore to change procedure without a change in statute.

The transfer of the blood to the container is best facilitated by allowing the syringe plunger to be pushed back up the barrel by the pressure increase of the blood from the first container before filling the second.

It is equally acceptable to insert another sterile needle into the membrane to allow pressure equalisation. If this is done the FME should record the presence of two holes in the membrane.

One anecdotal case had the accused specimen container sporting 16 holes whilst the "police" specimen had 1. Not all cases of interference would be as easy to spot as that, and it is good practice to record multiple perforation of the membrane.

It is sensible to develop a routine with RTA cases.

As the consent for a blood specimen is requested in front of a police officer who witnesses the response, there is no real requirement to have the consent to the simple transaction recorded in the clinician's record. If, however, the case is a more complex one involving examination then written consent should be obtained.

Many defences appear spurious and it helps to have developed a set notation for the record of the sampling, so that it can be seen that a detailed procedure was followed.

Recording:

- From which arm the sample was obtained.
- How much blood was obtained (if the syringe was not full).
- Who packaged the specimen.
- Was it "selotaped" and by whom?
- Was the accused given information about approved laboratories?
- The name of the authorised operator or police officer running the procedure.

and such like can all help.

---

r. "Where, at the time a specimen of blood or urine was provided by the accused, he asked to be provided with such a specimen, evidence of the proportion of alcohol or any drug found in the specimen is not admissable on behalf of the prosecution unless —

  (a) the specimen in which the alcohol or drug was found is one of two parts into which the specimen provided by the accused was divided at the time it was provided, and

  (b) the other part was supplied to the accused."

COMPLEX CASES

The simple cases involve those where the accused, having blown less than 50 µg of alcohol in 100 millilitres of breath (50 µg %), has claimed[83] to have it replaced with a blood or urine specimen.[s]

Other cases involve more difficult decisions.

Failure to provide a sample of breath - *the blood option*

This may happen at the roadside with the screening test and/or later with the definitive breath analysis device (BAD) in the police station.

A person failing to provide a specimen (of breath, blood or urine) is guilty of an offence under RTA **s7** (6) if there is no reasonable excuse for such failure.

This failure applies whether the request was under **s4** or **s5** of the RTA. The former making it an offence to drive if unfit so to do as a result of alcohol or drugs, and the latter for driving over the prescribed limit.

The constable has the option of whether the sample should be blood or urine (RTA **s7** (4)) unless a medical practitioner has cause to think a specimen of blood cannot or should not be taken. This choice leads to other interesting decisions which are dealt with below.

The constable can only opt for a blood (or urine) specimen at the police station, if it is not appropriate to use the BAD or one is not available or, it being a specimen under **s4**, he has been advised by a medical practitioner that the condition of the person required to provide the specimen might be due to some drug. (RTA **s7** (3) (c)).

Section 4 (5) of the RTA does state that the "person shall be taken to be unfit to drive if his ability to drive properly is for the time being impaired".

It can be seen however that there is **no** requirement of the police surgeon to prove impairment.

All the clinician has to do is demonstrate that there was a condition which could be associated with some drug. Alcohol can be a drug. The condition demonstrated could be caused by some other mechanism, eg hypoglycaemia, fatigue, but that is not an issue. However, though no case law has been found during the writing of this text by which a blood specimen was found to be inadmissable by virtue of the doctor's medical assessment being challenged to show a qualifying condition, it is appropriate for the FME to do a full examination and record all his/her findings and only proceed if a demonstrable condition is found. Nystagmus alone, even though found physiologically in a percentage of the pop-

---

s. Prescribed limits (July 1995) are

	Blood	80 mg %
	Urine	107 mg %
	Breath	35 µg %

ulation, could be due to a drug and therefore would seem to satisfy the requirements of the act.

What has been tested in the court is that the doctor must give an oral indication to the constable concerning the presence of a condition[84] and failure so to do may cause the specimen to be inadmissable.

There appears to be no requirement in the RTA for an accused to consent to a full examination, but there is also nothing in the act requiring the medical practitioner to do a full consensual examination before advising the police officer. It seems perfectly acceptable for the forensic clinician to observe the accused, record as much as possible of his/her observations and if there is a demonstrable condition satisfying the requirements, giving the advice anyway. The police surgeon must record accurately all the findings.

Failure to provide a sample of breath – *the breath option*

As has been mentioned on the previous page –

A person failing to provide a specimen (of breath, blood or urine) is guilty of an offence under RTA s7 (6) if there is no reasonable excuse for such failure.

There have been a number of cases whereby the lack of reception by the accused of the Statutory Warning has led to an acquittal. This could be due to lack of the warning being given at all[85] or for example not understanding the warning through a poor command of English.[86] Though these examples do not require medical input, it is conceivable that a clinical assessment may be required with this aspect in mind. This text will, however, concentrate on the areas where medical input is likely or necessary.

The question arises, when an accused fails to provide, as to what constitutes a "reasonable excuse". The police surgeon is often called in to assess this situation, but does not have to be.

A constable may determine the existence of a reasonable excuse as was proved with this example:

DPP *v* Pearman   Queen's Bench Divisional Court

before Lord Justice Lloyd and Mr Justice Waterhouse

Times Law Report 27 March 1992

Justices were entitiled, without having heard any medical evidence to find that shock combined with inebriation which rendered a defendant physically incapable of providing a breath specimen for analysis could amount to a reasonable excuse for failing to provide a specimen. This was held to be so in this case even though the accused had provided the first sample but failed on the second.

Reference was made to a previous judgment by Lord Justice Glidewell in *Grady v Pollard* ([1988] RTR 316, 323) who had said "Such evidence will normally be the evidence of a medical practitioner, but it need not be................."

Later in the substantive judgment however, Lord Justice Lloyd had added that this was not to say the justices should be gullible. The fact that a defendant was drunk, under stress or trying his hardest was not sufficient to be found a reasonable excuse. It was pointed out that the facts in this case went further.

This case of course does not say that a constable may determine the excuse was unreasonable without medical opinion.

A further case (Young *v* DPP)[87] held that intoxication was a reasonable excuse for failure to provide a sample of breath and did satisfy the requirements for requesting a laboratory sample (ie blood or urine).

It is likely that inadequate breath will be the commonest circumstance encountered.

Other conditions such as facial or dental injuries could well provide obvious cause of failure. As acute injuries sufficient to present problems are likely to be in hospital, then no specimen of breath will be requested and a laboratory test will be required subject to the medical practitioner in immediate charge of the accused's care does not object on grounds that the provision of such a specimen would be prejudicial to the proper care and treatment of the patient (RTA **s9**).

Obstructive airways disease is probably the only regular condition encountered.

Papers have been published on this subject.

Morris and Taylor,[88] having examined 5 accused and having performed tests on two intoximeters maintained that the requirement for 1.5 litres of air at 10 litres/minute (l/min), could be difficult for some patients to attain without adequate instruction and practice. One of the patients pleaded guilty; of the other four all had some clinical condition:- Obesity with angina and cardiomegaly; Ankylosing spondylitis; Asthma; Glottic closure with respiratory dyspraxia.

The contention was that each should have had the option of a laboratory specimen instead. As it was all four where acquitted of failure to provide a specimen of breath without reasonable excuse on the basis of the clinical material offered by the authors.

It can be seen that the police surgeon must have an open mind before stating that an accused did not have a reasonable excuse, and therefore not proceeding to a laboratory sample.

Work has been done on lung function. In the first paper[89] it was concluded that the most suitable measurements for determining an individual's capability to use a BAD were Forced Expiratory Volume in one second (FEV_1) and Forced Vital Capacity (FVC).

The conclusions were that:

1 Subjects with an

  1.1 FEV_1 of less than 2.0 litres and an

  1.2   FVC of less than 2.6 litres

were generally unable to use a BAD.

2 Ideally a spirometer should be available for use at the time of the breath alcohol test.

It was acknowledged that as spriometry is effort dependent, it will still be necessary to assess the degree of genuine effort being made.

The second paper by Gomm *et al*[90] looked at healthy people of small stature and their ability to use a BAD.

The conclusions in this case were that:

1 Subjects with a height of less than 5' 5" and an

  1.1 FEV_1 of more than 2.31 litres or

  1.2   FVC of more than 2.61 litres

should be able to satisfy the requirements of the test instruments.

It was also noted, in this work, that healthy people with a Peak Expiratory Flow Rate (PEFR) of greater than 330 l/min should be able to use the BAD.

The conclusion from these papers is that no accused should be deemed by a clinician not to have a reasonable excuse without spirometry readings, or in the case of a healthy person, a PEFR record which satisfies the criteria set by these papers.

Micro spirometers are available which can be easily carried in the medical bag.

A further point of note is that the constable may decide there are medical reasons for the non-provision of breath, such as the person's size, and require blood *even though the subject has denied that such reasons exist*.[91]

Failure to provide a sample of blood

As many of the blood samples arise from the accused's option,[83] they represent borderline cases of between 40 µg% and 50 µg% on breath analysis. The prescribed limit is 35 µg%.

Two matters acrue from this.

Firstly the police surgeon should not dally in arriving and completing the procedure. 45 µg% breath alcohol concentration represents about 102 mg% Blood Alcohol Concentration (BAC). If the accused metabolises alcohol at the average rate of about 15mg% /hour, a delay of just over 1½ hours could result in the sample being below the prescribed limit. If, on arrival the accused wished to reject a blood sample on the basis of a needle phobia, it may take 30 minutes to assess whether that was reasonable, and even if rejected, time has been used up. If accepted another hour could pass before the second of the two urine samples is legitimately obtained.

Secondly the analysis may need to be processed a number of times, particularly if close to the 40 µg% threshold, and the Home Office Laboratory will need as much blood as possible, preferably nearly 3 ml which is half that of the syringe in the RTA kits.

The answer to the first is easy – the FME should attend as soon as possible, and if other clinical duties (the police surgeon rarely being contracted or paid to give a dedicated service) prevent that, communication of this to the responsible police officer may give the latter the opportunity to find an alternative forensic clinician.

The second gives rise to a further decision.

The RTA requires the accused to **provide** a specimen (**s7** (1)(b)). Willingness to provide does not seem to be the issue. This reflects on the venesection. If the police surgeon attempts a venepuncture but fails, the attempt could, in theory, be made repeatedly until successful or until the medical practitioner advises the police officer under RTA **s7** (4) that in his/her opinion there are medical reasons why a specimen of blood cannot be taken. If a small sample is obtained and the volume is less than that on which the laboratory can perform an appropriate analysis (not less than 1ml[92] making a minimum of 2ml needed to be divided) a satisfactory sample has still not been obtained, and that sample must be discarded (see footnote page 140) and another one attempted or the same advice given as if no blood had been obtained at all.

In the case of analysis for drugs, obviously the laboratory need as much blood as possible. The RTA states in **s15**(5) "where...... he asked to be provided with a specimen". This relates to the accused being entitled to a specimen, the sample having been divided. The temptation to ask before splitting the sample, whether the accused wants his entitlement, or giving the accused a selected smaller volume in his specimen, should be avoided. The division of the sample should produce two parts both of which must be of a quality and quantity to be capable of analysis.[93]

A further issue arises if the accused complains of suffering from a condition which would be a reasonable excuse for not providing a blood specimen. Needle phobia is the obvious one.

NEEDLE PHOBIA

This subject is addressed particularly as experience has shown it to be a not uncommon excuse. Whether reasonable or not is now discussed.

The substantive case in this is :-

Regina v Lennard [1973] RTR 252

In this trial, the convicted person Michael Lennard had proposed that consuming a bottle of brandy after he had ceased to drive was a reasonable excuse for failing to provide a sample.[t] The evolution of the case was unusual and much of the trial and appeal related to procedure in law and is not relevant here.

However Lawton, Scarman and Phillips who heard the appeal did address the subject of reasonable excuse and produced the test by which excuses are now judged thus :-

" In our judgment no excuse can be adjudged a reasonable one unless the person from whom the specimen is required is physically or mentally unable to provide it or the provision of the specimen would entail a substantial risk to his health."

How this related to needle phobia became a judgment in 1974.

In Regina v Harding [1974] RTR 325, the Court of Appeal with Lord Widgery, Stephenson and Willis the conviction of failing to provide a specimen was quashed.

The judgement stated that the Regina v Lennard test was a good working rule and was satisfied in this case, but that " No fear short of a phobia recognized by medical science to be as strong and as inhibiting as, for instance, claustrophobia can be allowed to excuse failure to provide a specimen for a laboratory test, and in most if not all cases where the fear of providing it is claimed to be invincible the claim will have to be supported by medical evidence".

Thus it will come to pass that a police surgeon may have to assess an accused as to whether a needle phobia is a true phobia or, as was expressed in a further case[94] did the accused genuinely suffer from an " invincible repugnance to any use of the needle".

Naturally a history as to length of time of needle phobia needs to be taken. Other factors may help decide

- Do they travel abroad ? if so do they have travel vaccinations?
- Do they have dental treatment without local anaesthetic?
- Have they got pierced ears (or any other part of their anatomy)- how long have they had them?
- Have they got an obstetric history, did they have injections during that?
- Have they had treatment for the phobia?

---

t. The relevant statute then was the Road Safety Act 1967 s3 (3)- the words being the equivalent of RTA s7 (6) today.

An examination should be performed (with appropriate consent as with the history above) to look for signs of needle marks. These can be not just illicit "tracks", but GP tests, blood donation etc.

The physician can then make an informed decision as to whether the urine option is viable. Accepting the patient's word without checking may allow the accused to delay the proceedings long enough to affect the assay if urine is obtained. The FME has a duty to make a clinical decision.

IMPAIRMENT

There is one area in which the police surgeon may have to make an assessment of impairment. This arises from **s10** of the RTA which relates to the detention of an individual in the police station after they have been required to provide a specimen. Such a person may be detained at a police station until it appears to the constable that "were that person then driving or attempting to drive a motor vehicle on the road, he would not be committing an offence under section 4 or 5 of this Act".

Subsection (3) of this section states thus:-

" A constable must consult a medical practitioner on any question arising under this section whether a person's ability to drive properly is or might be impaired through drugs and must act on the medical practitioners advice."

Thus any examination performed under this section of the RTA demands a different assessment from **s7** (3)(c) as discussed above (see page 142). This is a forensic examination and appropriate consent is needed.

Such an examination should be most comprehensive and include a:

- General examination
- Spatio-temporal awareness assessment
- Demonstration of locomotor ability and balance
- Eye movement and co-ordination
- Demonstration of cognitive function

for more details of examination see page 81.

13

APPENDICES

APPENDIX 1a – Example of author's record chart, front

Dr. Stephen P. Robinson
Surgery:-277 Manchester Road, West Timperley, Altrincham WA14 5PQ
Tel:-0161 962 4351

Name .... Address ....

D.O.B. ....

● ●

I consent to a medical examination, including the taking of samples, if appropriate on myself
or/my ....
in connection with/ allegations of ....
as explained to me by Dr. Robinson.

I also consent to the consultation/examination :-
    a) being recorded in writing/audio/video
    b) involving the use of photographs which may be used in teaching
    c) findings being disclosed to the police/ social services/other ....

I also understand that anything I tell the doctor may have to be produced and declared if so ordered by a court.

Signed........................... Date ....

WITNESS
Signed........................... Date ....
(name / address / relationship of witness)
....

I confirm that I have explained the purposes of the "examination"
Signed........................... Date ....

APS SPS TMC 277 145 OTHER ....

OAPA 47-/20+ SOA DEATH Susp Y/N FTBD FTBI CONTAINER RTA S4/S5/? MHA

Disposal:- Remain/ Remove custody elsewhere/ Release/ Refer Hospital- Cas/ XR/OP/ Domi

ResponsibleOfficer............... ReportingOfficer/Operator ....

Fee
    Statement   Mileage
                  Date of::
Fee2 (hour/sub visit)

APPENDIX 1b – Example of author's record chart, back

PMSH

    S.H. Tobacco

        Alcohol

        Drugs

        Marital Status

        Employment

OE

General Findings

P	**BP**	**Facies**	**Nails**	**Gooseflesh**

RS   Air Entry

         Adventitiae

         Trachea

         P.N.

HS   I   II

         Murmurs

         JVP

ENT

ABD

CNS   Pupils   PERLA

          Fundi

APPENDIX 1c – Chart 1 Body A-P

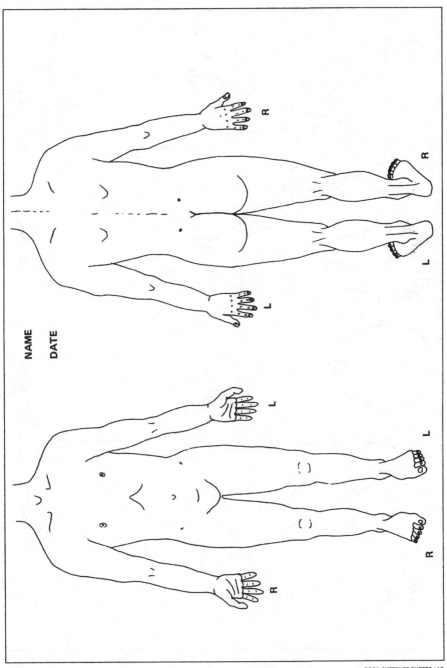

NAME

DATE

R

R

L

L

L

L

R

R

APPENDIX 1c – Chart 2 Body lateral

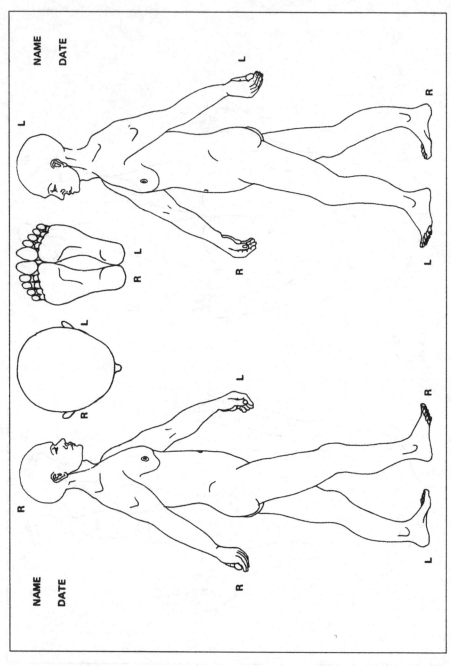

BODY SKETCHES SHEETS 2AB
©ASSOCIATION OF POLICE SURGEONS GREAT BRITAIN / BARBARA TYLDESLEY

APPENDIX 1c – Chart 3 Head

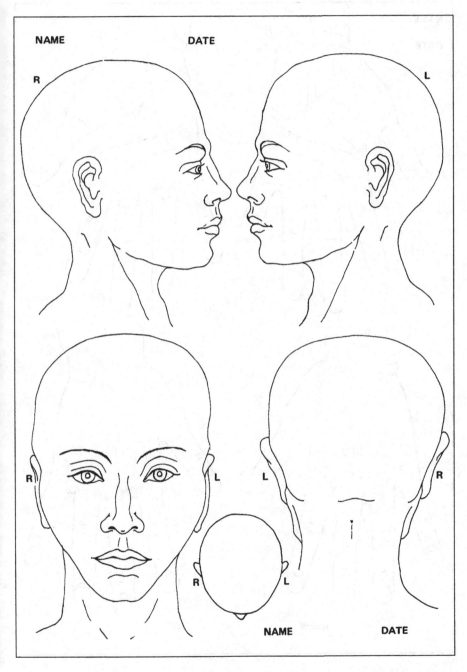

155

APPENDIX 1c – Chart 4 Hands

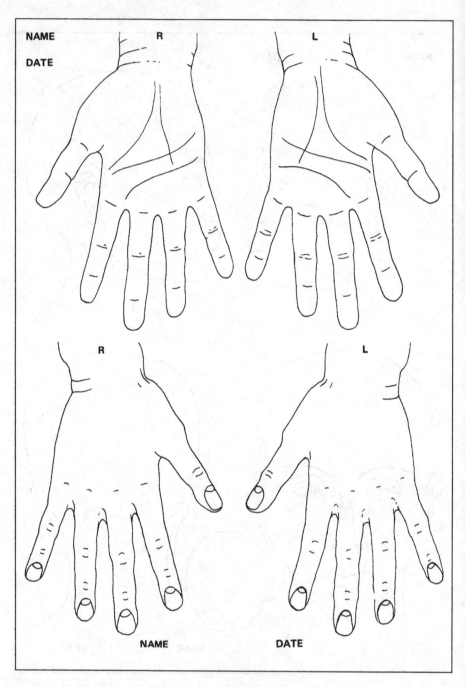

NAME

DATE

R   L

R   L

NAME   DATE

BODY SKETCHES SHEETS 4AB
©ASSOCIATION OF POLICE SURGEONS GREAT BRITAIN / BARBARA TYLDESLEY

APPENDIX 1c – Chart 5 Genitals

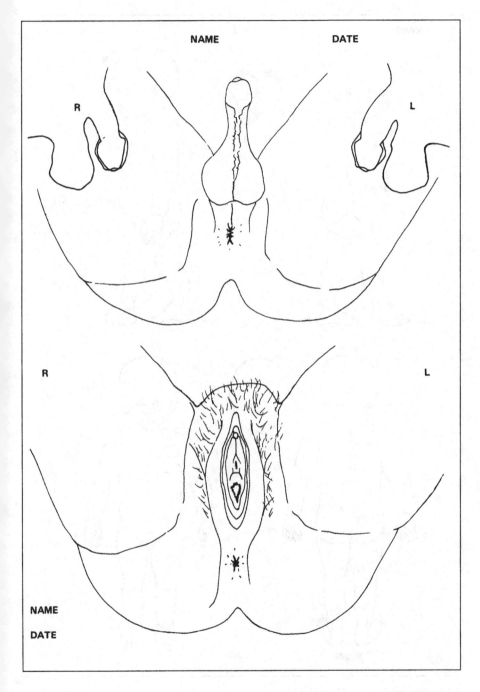

157

APPENDIX 1c – Chart 6 Child

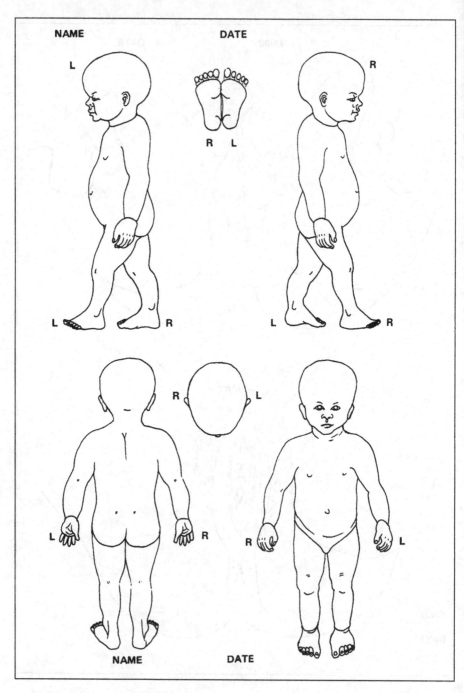

APPENDIX 1d – Example of simple record sheet, front

FORENSIC CLINICIAN GENERAL MEDICAL RCORD

Drs Name

Name .... Address . . . .

....

D.O.B. ....

I consent to a medical examination, including the taking of samples, if appropriate
on myself

or/my . . . .

in connection with/ allegations of

as explained to me by Dr.Robinson.

I also consent to the consultation/examination :-
   a) being recorded in writing/audio/video
   b) involving the use of photographs which may be used in teaching
   c) findings being disclosed to the police/ social services/other . . . .

I also understand that anything I tell the doctor may have to be produced and
declared if so ordered by a court.

Signed   . . . . , Date . . . .

WITNESS

Signed   . . . . , Date . . . .

(name address /relationship of witness)

. . . .

I confirm that I have explained the purposes of the "examination"

Signed   . . . . , Date . . . .

Location of examination. . . . .

Reason for examination . . . .

Disposal:- . . . .

ResponsibleOfficer. . . . . ReportingOfficer/Operator. . . . .

Fee
          Statement   Mileage
                                      Date of::
Fee2 (hour/sub visit)

159

APPENDIX 1e – Example of simple record sheet, back

PMSH

S.H.   Tobacco
            Alcohol
            Drugs
            Marital Status
            Employment

P

BP

Facies

Nails

Gooseflesh

RS

            Air Entry
            Adventitiae
            Trachea
            P.N.

HS

            Murmurs
            JVP

ABD

CNS

Pupils

PERLA

Fundi

NOTES

            DRUGS

APPENDIX 2 – Consent Form

Dr.Stephen P. Robinson

Address can be inserted here, either home, practice or local police station address

Name .... Address . . . .

....

D.O.B. ....

I consent to a medical examination, including the taking of samples, if appropriate on myself

or/my . . . .

in connection with/ allegations of

as explained to me by Dr.Robinson.

I also consent to the consultation/examination :-
   a) being recorded in writing/audio/video
   b) involving the use of photographs which may be used in teaching
   c) findings being disclosed to the police/ social services/other . . . .

I also understand that anything I tell the doctor may have to be produced and declared if so ordered by a court.

Signed   . . . . Date . . . .

WITNESS

Signed   . . . . Date . . . .

(name address /relationship of witness)

. . . .

I confirm that I have explained the purposes of the "examination"

Signed   . . . . Date . . . .

APPENDIX 3a – Drug misuse database form

IN CONFIDENCE: Please read notes on reverse

NORTH WEST DRUG MISUSE DATABASE
Local Monitoring of Problem Drug Use
Telephone Enquiries: 061-798 0544

and *NOTIFICATION OF DRUG ADDICTION*
Misuse of Drugs Act, 1971

Telephone Enquiries: 071-273 2213

Health Authority Code: **P** **1,8**
Home Office Code: **1,7**

For Database use Only:
Ref:
Date in:

Complete as much as you can of this form for every patient whom you attend who has a drug problem of any kind. The notification part of the form should only be sent to the Home Office if the person is notifiable. Use BLOCK LETTERS and a Ball Point Pen. Guidelines on reverse.

Details of Patient

First Name(s) | Last Name
Alias/Maiden Name (Delete)

Address | Date of Birth | Male ☐ Female ☐
Postcode | NHS No.
Ethnic Group

Employment: Present or last occupation
Employed ☐ Unemployed ☐ How long unemployed?

Referral From: Self ☐ GP ☐ Probation ☐ Family/Friend ☐
Psychiatrist ☐ Drug Team ☐ Other, specify

Notification: Is this person notifiable in accordance with the Misuse of Drugs Act 1971? Yes ☐ No ☐
If so, state which drug(s)

Drug Profile Past Month: include each drug used, prescribed or not *(if drug-free list significant prior use)*

	DRUG NAME	PRESCRIBED OR NOT Yes/No/Both	HOW OFTEN (times per day/wk/month)	HOW MUCH (quantity or cost per session)	ROUTE	DURATION (of this drug episode)	AGE OF 1st USE
MAIN DRUG							
DRUG 2							
DRUG 3							
DRUG 4							
DRUG 5 /alcohol							

Is person drug free? Yes ☐ No ☐ If Yes, how long? (See reverse)
Injected in past month? Yes ☐ No ☐ Ever injected? Yes ☐ No ☐
Shared needle/syringe in past month? Yes ☐ No ☐ Ever shared? Yes ☐ No ☐

Action Planned

Plan at onset: Nil action ☐ Planned O/P treatment ☐ Planned I/P treatment ☐ Further appointment ☐
Referred on ☐ specify where
Liaison with ☐ specify who/where

Prescribing plan: Nil ☐ Non-opiate drugs ☐ specify which
Methadone ... DTF ☐ or other forms, specify
Other opiates ☐ specify

Anticipate duration of prescribing (write NK if not known) Is this a reducing dose? Yes ☐ No ☐ Don't know ☐

Prescriber, if not yourself: GP ☐ Psychiatrist ☐ Drug Team Doctor ☐ Other

Details of Reporting Doctor

Name:

Patient seen in/at/by: General Practice ☐ Hospital Outpatient ☐ Hospital Inpatient ☐ Police Surgeon ☐
Prison Med. Service ☐ Other, specify

Treatment Centre/ Hospital/Practice: Name & Address
Postcode | Tel: | Date Seen

▶ This is your copy to retain

Drug Research Unit (University of Manchester) 061-798 0544
© Crown Copyright
Form 1990/3 M

APPENDIX 3b – Drug misuse database members

DATABASE USER GROUP MEMBERS
(as at June 1995)
Those marked with an asterisk use the same database form

North West RHA　★ Dr Michael Donmall Director Drug Misuse Research Unit Kenyon House Prestwich Hospital Bury New Road Prestwich Manchester M25 7BL	North Thames RHA　★ Arun Sondhi Database Officer The Centre for Research on Drugs and Health Behaviour 200 Seagrave Road London SW6 1RQ	South Trent RHA　★ Ian Ball South Trent Drug Misuse Information Systems Officer Drug Misuse Database Drury House 50 Leceister Road Narborough Leceister LE9 5DF
Anglia & Oxford RHA　★ Sharon Withnell Regional HIV & Drugs Offficer & Oxford Drug Database Anglia & Oxford RHA Old Road Headington Oxford OX3 7LF	Scottish Health Service Elaine Buist Statistician Information and Statistics Division Scottish Health Service Room BO23, Trinity Park House South Trinity Road Edinburgh EH5 3SQ	North Trent RHA　★ Anna Sefton/Stuart Bolton Drug Database Officer Rockingham Drug Project 117 Rockingham Street Sheffield S1 4EB
South Thames RHA Richard Goldfinch Centre for Addiction Studies Division of Addictive Behaviour St George's Hospital Medical School Cranmer Terrace, Tooting London SW17 0RE	South Thames RHA　★ Richard Hanstock Information Manager Substance Misuse Directorate Herbert Hone Clinic 11 Buckingham Road Brighton BN1 3RA	Welsh Health Common ★ Services Authority Sue McGuirk (Temp) Statistical Directorate CP2, Welsh Office Cathays Park Cardiff CF1 3NQ
North West RHA　★ Andrew Jones Senior Research Assistant Drugs & HIV Monitoring North West RHA Hamilton House Pall Mall Liverpool L3 6AL	South West RHA Barbara Boulton South West Regional Drug Problem Database Manager Ward 15 Blackberry Hill Hospital Manor Road, Fishponds Bristol BS16 1DD	South West RHA Gill Lillywhite Institute of Public Health Dawn House Romsey Road Winchester SO22 5DH
Northern & Yorkshire RHA ★ Jackie Murray Regional Drug and Alcohol Programmes Manager Northern & Yorkshire RHA Benfield Road Walker Gate Newcastle-upon-Tyne NE6 4PY	Northern & Yorkshire RHA Clare Pace Information & Operations Manager Leeds Addiction Unit 19 Springfield Mount Leeds LS2 9NG	West Midlands RHA　★ Marie Newman Drug Misuse Database South Birmingham RHA District Offices Vincent Drive Birmingham B15 2TZ

APPENDIX 3c – GMP fitness to be detained form

FORM 717

Greater Manchester Police
MEDICAL CERTIFICATE

Surname . . . .   Consec. No. . . . .

First Names . . . .

Date of Birth . . . .

Date . . . . Time . . . .

Where seen . . . .

TREATMENT ADVICE

The patient is suffering from

I recommend   . . . .

. . . .

. . . .

. . . .

. . . .

Fitness for Detention & Interview *(delete inappropriate items)*

The patient is Fit/Unfit to be detained and medical review should take place in . . . .
  hours/days

The patient is Fit/Unfit to be interviewed – An Appropriate Adult is/is not
recommended

If Unfit for Interview– Interview should not take place for . . . . hours & after
medical review

MEDICATION SCHEDULE

One Drug to a Line - If reducing course -use day column for reducing doses as per example	Date or mark "daily" if so required	**Breakfast** or delete & put time due below	**Lunch** or delete & put time due below	**Tea** or delete & put time due below	**Bedtime** or delete & put time due below		
		0830 Hrs	Hrs	1430 Hrs	Hrs	2200 Hrs	Hrs
Atenolol 50mg	daily	1					
Diazepam tabs 5mg	6/7/95			2		2	
- :: -	7/7/95	2		1		2	
- :: -	8/7/95	1		1		2	
- :: -	9/7/95	1		1		1	
If more than 6 drug lines are needed, use another sheet and tick the box here							
and mark the box here with the sheet number							

Doctor's Name. . . . .   Signature   . . . .

APPENDIX 3d – "Notifiable" diseases

NOTIFIABLE DISEASES

Cholera

Plague

Relapsing fever

Smallpox

Typhus

DISEASES WHICH ARE
REQUIRED TO BE NOTIFIED

Acute encephalitis	Ophthalmia neonatorum
Acute poliomyelitits	Paratyphoid fever
Anthrax	Rabies
Diphtheria	Rubella
Dysentery (amoebic or bacillary)	Scarlet fever
Leprosy	Tetanus
Leptospirosis	Tuberculosis
Malaria	Typhoid fever
Measles	Viral haemorrhagic fever
Meningitis	Viral hepatitis
Meningococal septicaemia	Whooping cough
Mumps	Yellow fever
Food poisoning	

APPENDIX 8a – GMP sexual assault - adult scheme

SCHEMATIC PRESENTATION OF GREATER MANCHESTER POLICE St MARY'S SEXUAL ASSAULT CENTRE

Health Care Staff at Centre

Forensic Clinicians –

Clinical Director (Dr Raine Roberts MBE)		
Team -	Female-	9
	Male-	5

All doctors have an honorary contract with the Central Manchester Healthcare Trust?(CMHT)
Centre Manager
Counsellors
Consultant Staff of CMHT provide services in Gynaecology
Venereology
Laboratory

Suite Design

Centre is suite of rooms with an Interview room designed to be comfortable and friendly but "trace evidence" compatible.
Examination room
Offices
Shower and toilet facilities
Lounge

Police Personnel

Senior Police Office as Liaison Officer.

Police Officers who are not part of dedicated team but who have specialist training including male and female SOCO photographers.

Patient Access

Patient complains to police ⇨ Force Ops contacts duty Dr ⇨ Dr provides examination at suite ASAP if alleged assault recent ⇨ Dr calls counsellor if latter not already there.
or

Patient presents at centre ⇨ Dr called (unless counselling only requested) ⇨ clinical data and specimens collected ⇨ formal complaint to police only if patient wishes.

Counselling continues in either case - continuation notes **not** considered part of contemporaneous record of allegation (therefore not classed as "unused material")

Patients Seen

1] All adults complaining of serious sexual assault

2] All children who have been allegedly subjected to stranger assault or rape, but not those where child protection issues are of primary concern and where abuse has been said to have been going on over a period of time.

APPENDIX 8b – GMP sexual assault – child scheme

SCHEMATIC PRESENTATION OF GREATER MANCHESTER POLICE CHILD ABUSE ORGANISATION

Each Police Division of GMP has a Family Support Unit (FSU).

FSU consists of specially trained officers who deal with domestic violence and child abuse.

Though divisionally organised they work without the police station and most have access to a well equiped child centred medical room.

Examinations may be carried out at these specialist centres, where video interview recording is available, or at St Mary's Sexual Assault Referral Centre, in hospital or GP surgeries if well enough equipped, and the environment is appropriate.

Examinations are never done in curtained cubicles in busy A&E suites, or ordinary medical rooms in police stations.

Medical staff who carry out this work consist of small group of appropriately trained and experienced police surgeons.

These clinicians also carry out examinations on behalf of, or with, social services, paediatricians and other doctors.

Call-out procedures are such that the calls usually come from the Force Operations Room, but they can originate directly from FSUs, hospitals or social workers.

The forensic physician will also give advice to other professionals and carry out examinations at the request of other doctors and social workers which may enable an opinion to be given that an injury is or is not the result of abuse. In some cases this may avoid the need to refer the case to the police, but in the interests of good practice and the well-being of the child and family, GMP has agreed to remunerate the doctor in such cases exactly as for a police referral.?

LIST OF ACRONYMS

A.A.	Appropriate Adult	F.S.U.	Family Support Unit
A.H.R.A.	Access to Health Records Act 1990	F.V.C.	Full Vital Capacity
		G.M.C.	General Medical Council
A.I.D.S.	Acquired Immune Deficiency Syndrome	G.M.P.	Greater Manchester Police
A.P.S.	Association of Police Surgeons	G.P.	General Practitioner
		H.O.F.S.L.	Home Office Forensic Science Laboratory
A.S.W.	Approved Social Worker	I.L.E.A.	International League Against Epilepsy
B.A.C.	Blood Alcohol Cocentration		
B.A.D.	Breath Analysis Device	M.D.O.A	Medical Defence Organisation
B.M.A.	British Medical Association		
B.N.F.	British National Formulary	M.H.A.	Mental Health Act 1983
B.T.S.	British Thoracic Society	N.H.S.	National Health Service
C.D.	Controlled Drug	O.C.P.	Over the Counter Product
C.M.O.	Chief Medical Officer	P.A.C.E.	Police and Criminal Evidence Act 1984
C.N.S.	Central Nervous System		
C.P.S.	Crown Prosecution Service	P.C.A.	Police Complaints Authority
C.S.A.	Child Sexual Abuse	P.C.C.	Post Coital Contraception
C.S.F.	Cerebro Spinal Fluid	P.E.F.	Peak Expiratory Flow
D.P.A.	Data Protection Act 1984	P.E.F.R.	Peak Expiratory Flow Rate
E.C.G.	Electro Cardio Graph	P.I.I.	Public Interest Immunity
E.D.T.A.	Ethyline Diamine Tetra Acetic Acid	R.M.O.	Resident (Receiving) Medical Officer
E.E.G.	Electro Encephalo Graph	R.T.A.	Road Traffic Act 1988
F.A.G.I.N.	Forensic Academic Group in the North	R.T.R.	Road Traffic Reports
		S.I.O.	Senior Investigating Officer
F.E.V.	Forced Expiratory Volume	S.O.C.O.	Scenes of Crime Officer
F.L.R.A.	Family Law Reform Act 1969	S.T.D.	Sexually Transmitted Disease
		S.W.O.T.	Strengths, Weaknesses, Opportunities, Threats
F.M.E.	Forensic Medical Examiner		

REFERENCES

1. FHSL (94) 30Preservation, Retention. and Destruction of GP General Medical Services Records Relating to Patients
2. Civil Evidence Act 1968
3. British Medical Association Ethics Committee & Association of Police Surgeons.(1994) *Health Care of Detainees in Police Stations*. BMA House, Tavistock Square, London
4. s8 Family Law reform Act 1969
5. ibid (sub sect 3)
6. Margaret Brazier (1992) *Medicine, Patients and The Law*. Penguin (p341)
7. Children Act 1989 s 3 (5)
8. 17 being the age of "adult criminality" according to the Children and Young Persons Act 1969
9. Children Act 1989 s 8
10. Part 3 paragraph 76
11. AHRA 1990 s1. (1) (b)
12. AHRA 1990 s1 subsection 2
13. AHRA S4
14. AHRA S 5
15. The Misuse of Drugs (Notification and Supply to Addicts) Regulations 1973
16. Personal communication from Dr Margaret Stark re correspondence with Home Office, Addicts Index January 1994
17. The Public Health (Control of Disease) Act 1984 and The Public Health (Infectious Diseases) Regulations 1988
18. Button James T H 1994 *Communicable Disease Control-A Practical Guide to the Law for Health and Local Authorities*:-Public Health Legal Information Unit in association with Department of Health & Welsh Office
19. National Health Service (Venereal Diseases) Regulations 1974
20. The National Health Service Trusts (Venereal Disease) Directions 1991
21. Cowley R 1994 *Access to Medical Records and Reports. A Practical Guide* -Radcliffe Medical Press, Oxford
22. Aspects of the Police and Criminal Evidence Act 1984: Medical Care of Detained Persons- Dr. M.A.Knight dissertation for University of Wales LL.M
23. Neilson *v* Laugharne[1981] 1 All ER 829.
    Heir *v* Cmm of Met.Police [1982] 1 All ER 335.
    Conerney *v* Jackson [1985] Crim LR 234.
    Peach *v* Cmm of Met.Police [1986] 2 All ER 129.
    Makanjuola *v* Cmm of Met.Police (1989) NLJR 468-
24. PCA Triennial Review 1988-1991
25. R *v* Chief Constable of the West Midlands Police, ex parte Wiley.
    R *v* Chief Constable of the Nottinghamshire Constabulary, ex parte Sunderland
26. Hunter D, Bomford RR *Hutchinson's Clinical Methods* Bailliere Tindell & Cassell
27. Issalbacher KJ (Eds) *Harrison's Principles of Internal Medicine* McGraw Hill
28. Lecture notes on Evidence by Mr Paul Taylor, Barrister given at FAGIN formed a considerable basis for this section

29. Cross on Evidence 7th Ed. p42 -approved by the House of Lords in R *v* Sharp 86 Cr App R 274

30. Bird R (1983) *Osborne's Concise Law Dictionary* 7th Ed. Sweet & Maxwell, London

31. The Criminal Justice Act 1988 s23 d

32. The Criminal Justice Act 1988 s24

33. Home Office Circular 17/50

34. World Health Organisation. Gastaut 1973

35. Issalbacher KJ (Eds) *Harrison's Principles of Internal Medicine* 13th Ed. McGraw Hill

36. Porter RJ (1985) *Epilepsy - 100 Elementary Principles.* W.B.Saunders, Philadelphia

37. *British Natonal Formulary* (BNF)

38. Issalbacher KJ (Eds) *Harrison's Principles of Internal Medicine* 13th Ed. McGraw Hill

39. Woodhead M (Ed) (1993) *Thorax*; 48 Supplement S22 BMJ Publishing Group, London

40. Bannister R 1968 *Brain's Clinical Neurology* 6th Ed. Oxford Medical Publications

41. Taken from Potter JM (1968) *The Practical Management of Head Injuries* 2nd Ed. Lloyd Luke

42. McLaren RE, Ghoorahoo HI, Kirby NG (1993)-Skull X-Ray recommendations of the Royal college of Surgeons Working Party in Practice. *Archives of Emergency Medicine* **10**: 138-144

43. Rix KJB, Rix EL (1985) *Alcohol Problems A Guide for Nurses and other Health Professionals.* Wright. PSG

44. Brismar B, Engstrom A, Rydberg U (1983) Head Injury and Intoxication: A Diagnostic and Therapeutic Dilemma *Acta Chir Scand* **149**: 11-14

45. Plum F, Posner JB *The Diagnosis of Stupor and Coma* Ed. 3rd. FA Davies

46. Law Commission Report No 229 (1995) *Legislating the Criminal Code: Intoxication and Criminal Liability.* HMSO

47. Robins E, Gassner S, Kayes J, Wilkinson RH, Murphy GE (1959) The communication of suicidal intent: a study of 134 successful (completed) suicides. *American Journal of Psychiatry* **115**, 724-73

48. James IP (1967) Suicide and mortality among heroin addicts in Britain. *British Journal of Addiction* **62**, 147-228

49. Gelder M, Gath D, Mayou R (1991) *Oxford Textbook of Psychiatry* 2nd Ed. Oxford Medical Publications

50. Mental Health Act 1983, s1 (3)

51. Payne-James JJ, Keys DW, Jerreat PG (1995) Salivary alcohol measurement: use in clinical forensic medical practice. *Journal of Clinical Forensic Medicine* **2**: 41-44

52. Rogers D *et al* (1995) presentation at 44th Annual Conference of Association of Police Surgeons

53. Payne-James JJ, Keys DW, Dean PJ (1994) Prevalence of HIV risk factors for individuals examined in clinical forensic medicine. *Journal of Clinical Forensic Medicine* **2**: 93-96

54. Police and Criminal Evidence Act 1984 (s.60 (1)(a) and s.66) Codes of Practice. Code C 9.5

55. Wetli CV, Fishbaine DA (1985) Cocaine Induced Psychosis and Sudden death *Journal of Forensic Science* **3**: 873-880

56. Reay DT, Howard JD, Fligner CL, Ward RJ 1988 Effects of Positional restraint on Oxygen saturation and Heart Rate following Exercise; *American Journal of Forensic Medicine & Pathology* **9**(1) 16-18

57. 1988 Philosophy and Practice of Medical Ethics BMA

58. Police and Criminal Evidence Act Codes of Practice (Revised Edition)- C 9.2 & Annex E

59. Clarke MDB (1991) Fit for Interview? *The Police Surgeon* **40**: 15-18

60. Gudjonsson GH (1995) "Fitness For Interview" During Police Detention: A Conceptual Framework for the Forensic Assessment *The Journal of Forensic Psychiatry* **6**(1): 185-197

61. Gudjonsson GH (1992) *The Psychology of Interrogations, Confessions and Testimony* Wiley, Chichester

62. WDS McLay (Ed) 1990 *Clinical Forensic Medicine* Association of Police Surgeons Chapter 6

63. Personal communication Paul Williams Lion Laboratories

64. Robertson G, Gibb R, Pearson R (1995) Drunkenness among police detainees *Addiction* **6**: 793-803

65. Glaus RA (1975) Suggestibility in young drug dependent and normal populations. *Br J. Addict.* **70**: 287-293

66. Gudjonsson GH, Clare I, Rutter S (1994) Psychological characteristics of suspects interviewed at police stations: a factor-analytic study *Journal of Forensic Psychiatry* **3**: 517-525

67. Sigurdsson J, Gudjonsson GH (1994) Alcohol and drug intoxication during Police Interrogation and the Reasons why Suspects Confess to the Police; *Addiction: Nordic Journal of Psychiatry* **94**: 915-917

68. Nemitz T, Bean P (1994) The Use of the " Appropriate Adult" Scheme (A Preliminary Report) *Medicine, Science and the Law* **2**: 161-166

69. Police and Criminal Evidence Act (s.60(1)(a) and s.66)- Codes of Practice C 11.1

70. Langlois NEI, Gresham GA (1991) The Ageing of Bruises: A review and study of the colour changes with time; *Forensic Science International* **50**: 227-238

71. Fineron PW, Turnbull J, Busuttil A. (1995) Fracture of Hyoid Bone in survivors of attempted manual strangulation; *Journal of Clinical Forensic Medicine* 2 Suppl: 6

72. Roberts R (1994) Case Presentations FAGIN

73. Wilson E Personal communication from Newton M- Metropolitan Forensic Science Laboratory- Research on donor sperm- Unpublished

74. Memorandum of Good Practice on Video Recorded Interviews with Child Witnesses for Criminal proceedings (1992) HMSO

75. Hemplin S (1991) The Aplications of Ultra-violet Photography in Clinical Forensic Medicine; *Medicine Science and the Law* **21**: 215-222

76. Police and Criminal Evidence Act 1984; Codes of Practice D 5.1

77. Mead J, Bonmarito L (1949) Reliability of rectal temperature as an index of internal temperature *J Appl. Physiol*; **2**: 97-109

78. Knight B (Ed) *The Estimation of the Time Since Death in the Early Postmortem Period*, Edward Arnold, London

79. Bernard Knight (1992) *Forensic Pathology* (p84). Edward Arnold, London

80. Lecture to FAGIN by Dr John Kennaugh University of Manchester Department of School of Biological Sciences and Forensic Entomologist.

81. Robinson SP (1993) *Analysis of Mental Health Workload in Suburban Police Surgeon Practice* Unpublished

82. Chairman Dr John Reed (1992) *Review of Health and Social Services for Mentally Disordered Offenders and Others Requiring Similar Services* HMSO Cm 2088

83. Road Traffic Offenders Act 1988 s8 (2)

84. Cole *v* Director of Public Prosecutions [1988] RTR p224

85. Simpson *v* Spalding [1987] RTR 221

86. Chief Constable of Avon and Somerset *v* Singh [1988] 107

87. Young v DPP Queen's Divisional Court before Lord Justice Lloyd and Mr Justice Waterhouse; *Times Law Reports* 27 March 1992.

88. Morris MJ Taylor AG (1987) Failure to provide a Sample of Breath Alcohol for Analysis *Lancet* 1987; 1(8523): 37

89. Gomm PJ *et al* (1991) Study into the ability of Patients with Impaired Lung Function to use Breath Alcohol Testing Devices *Med. Sci. Law*.3: 221-225

90. Gomm PJ *et al* (1993) Study into the Ability of Healthy People of Small Stature to Satisfy the Sampling Requirements of Breath Alcohol Testing Instruments; *Med. Sci. Law* 4: 311-314

91. Webb *v* DPP [1992] RTR p299

92. Private communication HOFSL Chorley and the author

93. Personal communication Chief Crown Prosecutor Greater Manchester and Cheshire.

94. Regina *v* Harding [1974] RTR 325

INDEX

Printed in the United States
By Bookmasters